HEALING
LESSONS

Sidney J. Winawer, M.D., with Nick Taylor

Little, Brown and Company

Boston   New York   Toronto   London

FIRST EDITION

Library of Congress Cataloging-in-Publication Data
Winawer, Sidney J.
    Healing lessons / Sidney J. Winawer, with Nick Taylor. — 1st ed.
        p.   cm.
    ISBN 0-316-94509-9
    1. Winawer, Andrea — Health. 2. Winawer, Sidney J. 3. Stomach —
Cancer — Patients — New York (State) — New York — Biography.
4. Physicians — New York (State) — New York — Family relationships.
I. Taylor, Nick.   II. Title.
RC280.S8W56   1998
362.1'9699433'0092 — dc21
[B]   97-46996

10   9   8   7   6   5   4   3   2   1

MV-NY

Book design by Barbara Werden

Published simultaneously in Canada by
Little, Brown & Company (Canada) Limited

PRINTED IN THE UNITED STATES OF AMERICA

To Andrea, for the love given so
generously to us all.
And to Joanna, Jonathan, and Daniel, for continuing
the meaning of life for me.

Acknowledgments

MANY people are owed thanks in connection with the preparation of this book, the events that inspired it, and for being there when we needed them. To try to list them all is to risk inadvertent oversight, but not to try is to commit the greater sin of not expressing heartfelt gratitude.

Family has never been more important. To my children, thank you for your strength and love and for the many thoughtful suggestions about the book. Joanna's memory was crucial to my recall of the facts; Jonathan helped me sort out the emotional dynamics; and Daniel's presence was supportive during the writing. To my sisters, Hinda and Joyce, thanks for your emotional support, your companionship, and your comments regarding the manuscript. To my sister-in-law, Marsha, whose memories enriched the book and who suffered through several losses during this period of time, thanks for your closeness. My gratitude embraces Norbert, Bruce, and all your families.

Dr. Robert Kurtz was an anchor of stability and a pillar of quiet wisdom. He and Moshe Shike were absolutely indispensable to my getting through the period of Andrea's illness professionally and personally.

Dr. Ian Robins was unstinting with his time, his medical expertise, his always sensitive advice, and most important, his friendship; he was a messenger of hope. Dr. Alan Turnbull came through for Andrea with superb surgery, and Ephraim Casper was her outstanding and trusted oncologist. Drs. Jose Botet, Subhash Gulati, Steve Sternberg, John Mendelsohn, Zvi Fuchs, Murray Brennan, Jimmie Holland, Kathy Foley, Lloyd Old, Richard Rifkind, Marty Fleisher, Anne Zauber, and Ms. Nessa Coyle provided expertise, understanding, and warmth in equal measure. Dr. David Golde contributed helpful suggestions. Above all, Dr. Paul Marks provided keen wisdom, compassion, and generous support, and also increased my capacity for exploring new professional directions, and his wife Joan was a source of personal encouragement.

Many people are essential for the diagnosis and treatment of a single patient with cancer. I am indebted to the Memorial Sloan-Kettering Cancer Center x-ray, laboratory, operating room, and intensive care unit staffs; the library staff, administrative personnel, and countless others; and the nurses and doctors, who were outstanding in their skills and empathy. My own Gastroenterology and Nutrition Service and GI Endoscopy unit staffs were constantly supportive. Professional colleagues at home and around the world responded whenever I called.

Sandy and Maurice Steinberg, Judy Fineberg, Anne Eden, Don Lefft, Judy Lefft, Rabbi Harvey Tattelbaum, Cantor Bruce Rubin, Lillian Clyde, Shirley McLean, Sam and Peggy Weiss, Pat and John Kadvan, Peter Tom, Bob and Sue Rahn, Zara Nelsova, and Jim Hayes were — and are — parts of the definition of true friendship. And Barbara Rose's unflagging support receives my deep appreciation.

Bill Phillips gave the editorial advice that helped in large measure to define what this book became. His assistants, Peter Ogden and Nicole Hirsch, kept it on schedule. The agents Morton Janklow and Lynn Nesbit placed it in capable hands at Little, Brown.

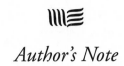

Author's Note

T HIS book does not prescribe a course of treatment. There are many different cancers, many different treatment options, and many different responses. Rather, it describes an approach to life and disease that can be beneficial. Patients should always consult with a qualified physician before embarking on a plan of treatment.

HEALING
LESSONS

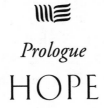

Prologue

HOPE

ANDREA and I listened on separate telephones as the smooth, seductive voice purred into our ears. She scribbled notes on a pad at the desk in our bedroom, where she sat. I watched her from the bed. Her eyes, shining with hope, flicked anxiously to mine. I frowned to show I was thinking.

Andrea had cancer. It had been three years since her diagnosis. The shock and fear we had felt at the time were mixed with an unusually bitter irony: in over twenty years at the Memorial Sloan-Kettering Cancer Center in New York, I had become a world authority on gastrointestinal cancers, and one of those was what she had. Since then, I had received almost daily lessons on what I didn't know.

As we confronted the limits of the conventional medicine I practice, we had moved into radical new territory. We found ourselves exploring new ground, not only medically, but in the emotional ties between us. At the beginning, I was her husband and lover, her provider, and the father of our children. Fulfilling each of those roles in the context of her cancer, I had become a different doctor. And a different man.

I frowned because the silken voice on the phone was spinning lies. They tempted Andrea to use a worthless weapon. But what the man was saying gave her hope. I had learned that hope was precious.

He was a "nutrition expert." We had sent him a sample of Andrea's blood. He had analyzed it and now was reporting the results.

"Your B.U.N. is slightly off," he said. "Eighteen. It should be sixteen."

He knew I was listening and that he didn't have to explain to me that B.U.N. was blood urea nitrogen. It is a measure primarily of kidney function. I knew that any reading up to twenty is perfectly normal. Andrea's kidneys weren't the problem.

"We can bring it in line with some special enzyme capsules," he continued smoothly. "Sixteen pills a day, four every six hours. Did I send you an order form?"

Andrea scribbled on the notepad and looked up to me for confirmation.

"He doesn't know what he's talking about," I started to say. Then I saw the hope in her eyes and kept quiet.

From the beginning, I had struggled with the same dilemma: where did the doctor stop and the husband and lover begin? The doctor was Chief of the Gastroenterology and Nutrition Service at Memorial Sloan-Kettering. I saw gastrointestinal cancers every day; indeed, I had devoted my professional life to their treatment and research. That Andrea had one — a neuroendocrine carcinoma of the stomach, to be precise — was plain cruel fate. Being a cancer specialist was one thing, being a cancer patient's spouse was something else. It changed everything. My doctor's certainties dissolved in a swirl of emotions. The most important, and also the most dangerous of these emotions, was hope. There was no way to deny it or deflect its power. My hope, as well as Andrea's, clung to every possibility.

That was the crazy thing. I really wanted to believe what the man on the phone was saying. I needed hope as much as she did. I loved her, and the prospect of losing her was more than I could bear. I knew he was talking garbage. I'm sure he knew I knew it, too. But he also knew

I would do anything to preserve Andrea's hope, and mine. It helped us keep fighting.

"The enzyme capsules will adjust your metabolism, a very slight correction," the "nutritionist" was saying. "That will help your body fight the cancer."

Until Andrea's cancer, I had underestimated the value of hope. Now it tugged at me. I thought, as the man spoke, If only it were true. We would dance in the streets. If Andrea could hope, I had to hope with her. I would lay aside my medical training, my instincts, my experience, as long as we could hope.

The conversation ended and we hung up the phones. "What do you think, Sid? It sounds good, doesn't it?" Andrea took an order form for the capsules from the desktop and held it out to me. There were blanks to order hundreds of pills costing hundreds of dollars. We were eligible for a special discount, since I was a doctor. The man not only was seducing Andrea with false possibilities, he was patronizing me.

I looked at her, heartstruck. Successive rounds of chemotherapy had taken her hair, clump by dark, wavy clump. Now she was bald, hairless over her entire body, and still her beauty made me ache.

"I don't know, Andrea. There's no evidence that it will help. But there's no evidence against it, either. We don't know everything in medicine. Maybe he's right. Maybe he has insight we don't have. It's happened before."

"It has, hasn't it." She brightened, and I breathed more easily. I took the capsule order form from her outstretched hand.

Andrea had survived as long as she had in part by defying medical convention. She didn't dismiss it entirely, but she integrated conventional treatments with approaches that some doctors dismissed and many disapproved. I had been among the naysayers, but I had become a believer. I saw that patients working with doctors had the potential to revolutionize medicine today and in the future. I saw the impact of her self-empowerment. I saw her mind act to heal her and make her well. I felt the strength of faith and prayer. She taught me new lessons in healing.

The last three years of anguish, pain, and fear had educated and transformed us and our family. They vibrated with discoveries. Our life together was richer. I was learning to be a better husband and father. I was learning to be a better doctor, learning from her that conventional medicine, the kind I had practiced all my life, did not hold all the answers. She helped me learn that doctors do not heal alone, without learning from the patients they treat.

Now, I confronted the risks of that approach. Andrea held the reins. She was empowered to make informed and sometimes radical decisions. A good doctor would take advantage of her wish to believe. A charlatan would exploit it for gain, as the enzyme capsule man was doing. I struggled to find the line between hope and doubt, knowing that if you believe in miracles, sometimes they occur.

I still was learning that the miracle you hope for is not always the miracle that you receive.

Chapter

1

NEW YORK CITY, December 31, 1990.
New Year's Eve was a light day because of the approaching holiday, not the usual twelve hours. I had spent the day at the hospital, talking over patients' problems with the fellows-in-training who had seen them first, making rounds, reviewing charts and making entries, then retreating to my office to catch up on the inevitable paperwork demanded of a service chief. I dictated some letters and made notes for a lecture I was to deliver in two weeks to other specialists at a seminar in Boston. I headed home early, about seven.

When I got home, Andrea already had started preparing for the evening. The children — Daniel, Jonathan, and Joanna, in order from oldest to youngest — all were old enough to attend New Year's Eve parties of their own. We were going to our regular New Year's get-together. It was a group of old friends and fellow music lovers, hosted by an opera singer and her husband. We always had fun, and I looked forward to it.

Andrea was in a talkative mood. She was usually more talkative than I. She was a better listener, too, a quality that endeared her to everyone she knew. Andrea was a "people person" whose interest and attention inspired others to confide in her. Now, the old year sliding toward the new was making her reflect and look ahead.

"Think of it, Sid," she said, holding up an outfit and surveying its effect in the mirror of our bedroom. "Another year, and we'll be looking forward to Joanna's high school graduation. Jonathan will be halfway through Columbia. Daniel's going to find his way, I'm sure of it. And then . . ." She raised an arm dramatically. "Weddings and grandchildren, who knows?"

I looked ahead and saw a life without tuition payments, cutting back on work, a time when she and I could travel more together. The thought made me smile. We had more money than my parents had ever dreamed of having. We wanted for nothing. But my choice of academic medicine, with its emphasis on teaching and research in addition to private practice, meant there were some financial limits.

"What do you think?" she asked me.

The dress she held in front of her was black, simple, and attractive. Andrea devoted a lot of time to looking good. "I like it," I said.

"I'll wear a bright scarf with it." She pulled the dress over her head and spun around, a movement of the dancer she once had wanted to be. "Zip me, please." She tilted her head and looked back at me over her shoulder. Her movements always had a touch of drama. The twist of her long neck was as elegant as a swan's. Her hair had the color and the gloss of ebony.

I drew the zipper up along the stark ridge of her backbone. Her ribs fanned out to each side. The bones were too stark, too exposed, the result of her chronic anorexia. She didn't eat her food, she pushed it around on the plate. It drove me crazy sometimes, watching her. Years of therapy hadn't made much difference. All of us had been in therapy, separately and together, trying to identify and solve problems that percolated under the surface of our lives. Sometimes it seemed as if we couldn't move without our therapist's advice. It also seemed, sometimes, as if we were lost in a funhouse, each mirror providing a new image to which we had to reorient ourselves. For the kids and me, it was less frequent, but Andrea had been going to sessions for nine years. Lately, she had been saying that she was ready to get better. She was ready to tackle and resolve the underlying issues. Maybe she was right. Maybe we were about to turn the corner. The thought of losing the therapy bills didn't make me unhappy.

"I hope you're right," I said.

"Sidney Jerome." She pouted, then smiled, and placed a hand against my cheek. "Be an optimist. We have so much to look forward to."

My cheek tingled from her touch. I drew her against me and snuggled into the curve of her neck. My "spot," she called it. I felt we connected there.

A few minutes later, we left for the party.

New Year's was never a big event for me. It never moved me to make resolutions. Resolutions imply the need to change. Most people never keep them. I always preferred to set goals and work toward them. I was in high school when I made it my goal to become a doctor. It seemed to me, a child of Polish immigrants in Brooklyn, that doctors were the wisest and most compassionate of people. The milkman, the kosher butcher, the strolling cops, even most of my teachers, were familiar and commonplace. But doctors knew the secret art of healing. They had knowledge the others didn't have. Nobody questioned them. They received respect and admiration, even awe. I wanted that respect and special knowledge. I wanted to know how to heal and make things right. I felt it was my destiny, and so I set my sights. My family didn't have much money; my father's income as a baker barely supported my parents, my sisters, and me, but I knew that I could make it. I studied, worked in my spare time, pushed my social life into the background, and followed the straight and steady path. And it had happened. Now I had the life I'd dreamed of: professional satisfaction, a beautiful family, a large apartment and a beach house, winter ski trips, nights at concerts and the opera. The problems that had taken us to therapy diminished none of that. When it came to New Year's Eve, I felt I didn't need to make new promises. It was hard work to keep the ones I'd made already.

The party, true to form, was warm and simple. We talked with our friends about our kids and our plans for the future. We ate from a buffet of pasta and salad. A couple sat down at the piano and entertained the group with show tunes as we sang along. As the hour ticked toward midnight, we all turned to the television tuned to the mass of people in Times Square. They were rowdy, happy, and expectant. The ball descended, and we clinked glasses to happiness, good health, and long lives.

The party broke up not long after midnight. Andrea and I were home in bed by one. Around one-thirty, she shook me awake. I woke instantly, the legacy of medical training. One sleepless week as a nervous intern waiting for calls, and then I learned to sleep at odd moments and wake up at a blink. Like most doctors, I retained the knack.

Our bed was under the window. The city's nighttime glow shone on the delicate features of her face. People often said she looked like Audrey Hepburn, a resemblance they found in her pert nose, wide mouth, full lips, and warm eyes. I was startled to see her grimacing with pain.

"Do we have any antacids?" she asked in a strained voice. "I think I'm having a little spasm here."

We always slept nude, and she lifted her breasts to show me the location of the pain. It was high in her stomach under her rib cage. She fanned a hand down, showing me that it radiated to her lower chest.

Andrea never complained, so I knew she was hurting. I got her an antacid tablet from the medicine cabinet in the bathroom. The pain subsided after she took it, and we went back to sleep.

An hour later, I felt her hand on my shoulder again. She was frowning and holding her stomach. I got her another antacid, wondering what she could have eaten, but again the pain subsided and we returned to sleep.

The third time, I woke up when she began to stir, before she touched me. The third antacid soothed the pain again, and again she fell asleep. She slept through the night this time, but I lay awake. A diagnostic alarm bell was ringing in my brain.

I WAS worried.

Worry was the one thing that interfered with my doctor's ability to sleep. I worried mostly about other people — Andrea, our kids, my patients. I worried about my parents when they were still alive. I had this need to be responsible and in control. I even felt responsible for the things I couldn't control, like the weather. "I'm really sorry it's raining. I feel so bad," I would tell people if they happened to visit us at our beach house on a washed-out weekend. I never quite believed them when they said, "Sid, it's not your fault." I had to take care of everybody and everything — to organize, arrange, protect, and heal. Being in control made things easier.

I managed and took care of everybody but myself. Because I was older than Andrea, and a man, I assumed that she would outlive me and could be a widow for years. I worried about what would happen to my family after I was gone. I worried about who would take care of Andrea and the children financially, so I made sure I had plenty of life insurance and investments. Now, lying beside her and listening to her steady breathing, running through the possibilities, I added Andrea's health to my list of worries.

"HOW do you feel?" I asked when she woke up in the morning.

"Just fine." She smiled and stretched like a cat in the daylight streaming through the window. The "spasms" of the night before were gone.

"Are you sure? Show me where it was again."

"It was just something I ate at the party. For goodness sake, stop worrying." She rose, slipped on a robe, and headed into the kitchen to make coffee.

I wanted to follow her suggestion. If I stopped worrying, we would have another comfortable, familiar morning, and we could go on with our lives. But I knew nothing she ate caused last night's pain. She had eaten, and drunk, hardly anything at all at the party, in keeping with her anorexia. I thought her pain was probably an ulcer. My next thought was, What kind of ulcer?

As a gastroenterologist, I knew most ulcers are benign. If properly treated, they're usually cured. When they're painful, antacids or food often produce quick improvement. Most benign stomach ulcers today are caused by anti-inflammatory drugs used to treat arthritis and various other musculoskeletal disorders — drugs such as Indocin, Motrin, and Advil. Andrea was taking none of these drugs. The other common kind of ulcer occurs in the duodenum, the first portion of the small intestine just below the stomach. These are almost always benign, and most of them, along with some stomach ulcers, are caused by a bacterial organism, Helicobacter, or *H. pylori,* that can inhabit the stomach. It irritates the cells that produce acid, stimulating acid flow that in turn causes the ulcer. *H. pylori's* discovery by an Australian doctor has revolutionized the understanding and treatment of ulcers, and a week or two of antibiotics usually gets rid of the bacteria.

I'll settle for that, I thought. But Andrea's pain had been high in the abdomen, and that was a warning signal. It was too high to be from either a benign stomach or a duodenal ulcer. I feared that, if she had an ulcer, it was malignant — stomach cancer.

I told myself I was overreacting, but statistics ping-ponged around in my brain. They were sobering. Gastric (stomach) cancer is the most common cancer worldwide, although it lags behind other forms of cancer in the United States. Lung, breast, and colon cancer each account for well over one hundred thousand new cases annually. Prostate cancer is virtually epidemic, with about three hundred thousand cases diagnosed each year. Stomach cancer accounts for just a fraction of those numbers. Still, over twenty thousand new cases are reported each year in the United States. It strikes more women than men. The patients are usually in their sixties or older. But I had seen enough cases in younger people to know that Andrea, who was forty-five, was not exempt. That she might be one of those twenty thousand was a chilling thought.

The smell of coffee beckoned the children from their rooms. One by one, Joanna, Jonathan, and Daniel appeared, picked up sections of the newspaper, looked in the refrigerator, poured coffee, disappeared again. The coffee's aroma seemed to sharpen my worry. Andrea's pain came on suddenly, as if from nowhere. That meant that if there was a stomach cancer, it had been present for some time. It had ulcerated and gone deep and irritated the pain fibers of the stomach wall. This was the con-

sistent, almost inevitable course of the disease. Her symptoms were a
red flag. They told me not to wait.

"Let's just be sure," I said, accepting the steaming mug she handed me.

"Sid, I had a pain, it's gone, let's just forget it."

I dropped the subject, and we lazed away the rest of New Year's Day.
We ate a late breakfast, and later went out to a movie and dinner with
the kids. At Louie's on Amsterdam Avenue, we chose one of the tables
on the open balcony so the five of us could have a cozy and private family dinner. Looking down at the other diners made me feel that we were
insulated from them and the world. The candlelight and conversation
gave a sense of closeness that wasn't always there now that the children
were older. When they were young we had spent hours on end with
them, especially at the beach house; I had driven them to elementary
school, and we had shared traditional Shabbat dinners on Friday
evenings before temple. As they developed lives of their own, we had to
create occasions for togetherness. Andrea had made our New Year's Day
movie and dinner a regular affair. The kids were important to her. All
too soon — now that Jonathan and Daniel both were in college, and
Joanna just eighteen months from high school graduation — they
would be scattered to the winds. But for the moment, the family was as
we both imagined. I felt happy as we sat around the table, but not entirely at peace. I had a gnawing feeling that something was not right.

The next morning, over Andrea's objections, I called for an appointment with one of my colleagues at Sloan-Kettering.

Bob Kurtz headed the gastrointestinal endoscopy unit in my service
at the cancer center. He was perhaps the closest of many close colleagues; we had seen and talked with each other almost daily for twenty
years, and I relied on his judgment. If there was bad news, I wanted to
hear it from him. Of course, you don't go to the doctor for bad news.
You go to hear that the problem is a minor one and that a few pills will
take care of it; otherwise, you might not make the appointment so
quickly. Andrea knew Bob and was comfortable with him. If it came to
that, they would form the kind of doctor-patient relationship that made
everything that followed easier.

"I'd be glad to see her," he said. "When does she want to come in?"
"Today."

He hesitated in surprise. Then he checked his schedule and picked a time. Andrea and I arrived together. Bob waved us to seats and sat back behind his desk. "What's wrong?" he said. "Sid said you wanted an appointment right away."

Andrea downplayed her symptoms. I kept the worst of my fears to myself, knowing that Bob was an excellent gastroenterologist and endoscopist, and a fine physician overall, serious and thorough, with good medical instincts. He would find out what, if anything, was wrong. I left while he took a medical history from Andrea and then examined her. He ordered blood drawn for routine tests. He called me back at the end of the examination.

"See," said Andrea triumphantly when I entered the room. "It was just something I ate." She looked to Bob for confirmation.

"We'll see what the blood tests show," he hedged. "But based on what she told me, it does sound like she just had an upset stomach."

Bob and I sat there in our white coats and looked at each other. His eyes were kind and intelligent, and they showed his concern that I wouldn't have asked for such a quick appointment if I hadn't been worried about something. We both knew, also, that friendship and emotional ties can push doctors toward a rosy outlook. Bob's friendship gave him a stake in the diagnosis. Doctors like to avoid treating family members and close friends for that reason. Emotional factors enter in. You don't want to bring bad news into the relationship, and so you sometimes shy away from the more serious possibilities. I was sure that Andrea had minimized her symptoms. Many patients do, and then take comfort when they hear what they want to hear from the doctor. An upset stomach was what we all wanted.

"What would you do if it were somebody else?" I asked him. If we were laymen, he would have thought I was an anxious, worrisome, overprotective spouse.

He glanced at Andrea. "I'd do an endoscopy," he said.

"Then do it."

Chapter

2

ANDREA made a face. For several weeks, she had resisted my suggestions that she get a checkup. She said she was tired, but the tiredness always disappeared after she had a productive therapy session. She had come to hear that it had been something she ate. Now, she was facing more diagnosis than she had bargained for. It occurred to me that perhaps she had resisted because she anticipated bad news.

Bob scheduled her for an endoscopy that Friday, January 4. She approached the appointment as an inconvenience.

On Thursday, I was in my office looking over some slides for a lecture when my secretary put through a call from home. The lilting West Indian voice on the phone was that of Shirley McLean, our housekeeper. She and Andrea were exceptionally close. Shirley brought her three sons to work with her when they were young, and Andrea opened our home to them. She and Andrea usually ate lunch together. They talked, and Andrea would play music, oldies but goodies that they both enjoyed, and they would dance together in the kitchen. This was the quality of Andrea that everyone loved. Shirley's voice was concerned.

"Doctor Sid, could you bring some gas pills home? We're eating lunch, and Andrea, she's sick. She's having gas pains."

"How often?"

"Oh, Lord, every fifteen minutes."

Gas pains. An upset stomach. The easy answers that keep people from seeing doctors until something is really wrong. My worry sharpened. But I hid my worry from Andrea when I got home that evening. Doctors often think of the worst possibilities, and I didn't want to alarm her. Also, as a doctor, I was used to spooning out information in easy-to-take doses.

Friday came. "What should I wear?" were Andrea's first words when she got up.

"Anything. Bob won't care."

But Andrea liked to look right for every occasion, even an endoscopy. Her closets contained clothes that were bright and fashionable, but simple. She chose a red skirt and a black sweater, set off by a scarf that was a swirl of colors. Joanna left for school. Jonathan got ready to go to the data entry job at Sloan-Kettering I had arranged for him during his winter break from Columbia. Daniel, also on winter break from college but not working, was still asleep when Andrea and I left for the hospital at eight.

Memorial Sloan-Kettering is huge. Its two major units, Memorial Hospital and Sloan-Kettering Institute, occupy an entire city block on New York's Upper East Side, between York and First Avenues, and 67th and 68th Streets. Nearly six thousand employees, including almost five hundred doctors and eight hundred nurses, work there. We entered through the back entrance on First Avenue. There's nothing about this simple portal, with its two sets of doors and security guard's station, that says "world-class cancer center." Most people go in the main entrance on York Avenue, but the back way was more convenient from home, and also closer to my office and the endoscopy unit. We nodded at the guard and went to the fifth floor of the outpatient building.

While my position at the hospital guaranteed that Andrea would have an unusual level of access to care — no better than other patients would receive, but more expeditious — she wasn't exempt from the preliminaries required of all patients. She filled out the usual forms with their questions about allergies to medication, past medical history, and prior procedures. Then she went to the women's locker room to change.

When she emerged, in a hospital gown, the sight shocked me. She had been shapely and sexy in her skirt and sweater; now, in the loose gown, she was without form. I had never thought until that moment how utterly and completely people give up their individuality and control when they become patients. They're told, "Sit here. Fill out these forms. Stick out your arm. Lie down. Open your mouth." They enter a world with a strange language and unfamiliar rules, in which they are no longer in control. They don't even have their clothes to provide identity. I saw that it was certainly humbling, probably frightening, and perhaps humiliating to be so totally under the command of others. My reaction spoke volumes about what patients sacrifice in dignity and self-esteem, and what I, as a doctor, had not seen quite this way before.

A nurse led Andrea to one of the endoscopy rooms. She would fasten electrocardiograph leads to Andrea's chest, wrap a blood pressure cuff around one arm, and place an oxygen monitoring clip on one finger. All patients getting intravenous sedation received this multi-tiered monitoring.

While this was going on, I entered a small, closed room with television monitors lined up along a shelf, each monitor connected to an endoscope in one of the four procedure rooms along the hall. Here in the control room, I would be able to see exactly what Bob saw as he performed the endoscopy.

Suddenly Bob pushed through the door, his long face grim. He held a computer printout that I recognized as blood test results.

"Sid, there's something going on," he said, tension straining his voice. "Her liver function is abnormal, and her hemoglobin is eight-point-eight."

"Eight-point-eight?" The figure stunned me. I didn't have to look at a chart to know it was 30 percent below normal, a striking abnormality. It indicated severe anemia. Andrea must have been bleeding from the stomach for several months, oozing only traces day by day that would have kept her from noticing the telltale signs — a darkening of her stool, for example. Her body would have compensated, producing no dramatic symptoms that could have been a warning.

I thought back again to those times during the past few weeks when she said she felt drained and tired. When she came home from her therapy sessions energized, talking about how good she felt, the fatigue seemed emotional and not physical. Now I wondered. For years, dating to the start of her therapy, Andrea had seemed to tire easily. It had been months since I tried to persuade our psychiatrist to recommend that she get a checkup and blood tests, but he dismissed the suggestion. So did she. When she finally had blood tests done by her gynecologist, the report came back marked "Lab accident. Repeat." She wouldn't go. Andrea was diligent about Pap smears and breast exams, but thought she was too young to waste her time with general checkups.

"I don't need to," she argued. "I feel fine. I get tired now and then, but there's nothing wrong with me that therapy can't cure."

Well, bleeding ulcers are cured every day. That's what I told myself as Bob left for the room where Andrea waited.

I envisioned the endoscopy procedure. I had done it myself thousands of times. Bob would administer Andrea sedation in an IV drip to get her ready. She would quickly doze off. Then, he would pass the endoscopy tube, no thicker than the average person's little finger, through a mouthpiece into Andrea's stomach by way of her esophagus. The flexible tube would light the stomach with thousands of fiber-optic threads and transmit the picture in full color to the monitors by means of a computer chip. The tube's open channel would allow a biopsy forceps and other fine instruments to obtain tissue samples, or bundles of laser-transmitting fibers to destroy growths. It was a procedure that seemed invasive only if you forgot what endoscopes had been like years ago. In my training I had manipulated rigid pipes of steel down the throats of patients who had to throw back their heads like sword swallowers to admit the instrument. Later, endoscopy tubes were part rigid and part flexible, and contained a series of tiny mirrors. Now, they were so flexible that you could tie them in a knot and still see clearly what was at the other end. Today's instrument was superior in every way. At $100,000, including all of its computerized components, it should have been.

The monitor flickered. Bob now had the endoscope entering Andrea's stomach. The view it provided was something like that of the inside of a cave or a mine shaft provided by the lamp on a miner's helmet. It is dark inside the stomach, but after a few puffs of air distend the stomach cavity, the light illuminates it quite well and brightly. Every tiny little spot can be seen clearly, even around curves. An ulcer appears as a small crater, usually with a grayish center. A tumor is a mound, sometimes with an ulcer in it. If the ulcer is bleeding, you can usually see the blood trickling from it. Sometimes the ulcers and tumors can be quite large and the blood flow extensive. The healthy stomach wall looks flesh-colored, with a hint of orange from the endoscope light, the healthy stomach lining fairly smooth with small longitudinal ridges. Nothing disturbs the orderly landscape. That is what we hoped to see, I in the control room and Bob on a monitor near Andrea's stretcher as he handled the instrument.

I watched the monitor with apprehension. The light in Andrea's stomach showed a healthy-looking stomach wall. I held my breath. Second by second, centimeter by centimeter, the light fell on healthy tissue. The scope passed through the pylorus, the valve that connects the stomach with the upper part of the small intestine. The intestinal lining pulsated with each heartbeat. Everything looked good. The light withdrew back into the stomach.

Now Bob maneuvered the scope back on itself, as if a snake dangling by its tail was raising its head. In retroflexion, the light shines up, sweeping the area of the stomach that is hard to see on the way down. We were almost home. Almost. Then something new appeared on the monitor. The light found and centered on a raised mass, ulcerated and bleeding at the center. I stared. Something was wrong with the monitor. It was receiving pictures from a different endoscope, not the one in Andrea's stomach.

I went numb and cold. My chest tightened. I literally felt the floor shift under my feet and I grabbed the counter as my knees buckled. The tumor was big, and clearly malignant. Andrea, my God, no! I wanted to erase the picture from the monitor and step into the hall, where I would emerge, like Alice from the well, back into reality.

Bob entered the control room and found me still gripping the counter and staring at the now-blank screen. I turned my face to him. He took one look and embraced me.

"I'm sorry, Sid," he said as he patted me gently on the shoulder. "Which surgeon?"

"Turnbull." My voice sounded far away, as if it were someone else speaking.

Questions flew at me, the automatic result of years of training. Two stood out. How extensive was the cancer? And what was its pathology type?

We paged Dr. Alan Turnbull, whose surgical specialty was gastrointestinal cancer. He was an excellent surgeon, one of many at Memorial Sloan-Kettering. Andrea knew and liked him, a recommendation in itself because her judgment about people was invariably on target. And he was aggressive, not likely to back off if the operation turned difficult.

She awoke in the recovery room to find the three of us standing at her bedside. She looked from face to face, sensing through her sedation that the gathering of doctors meant bad news. I took her hand while Bob told her. "Andrea, we've found a tumor. That's all we know right now. I've ordered some more tests to check it out further."

The grogginess muted her reaction, but the aftereffects of anesthesia did not keep the alarm from her eyes. Barely able to focus them, she looked at me for reassurance, some sign that would tell her I could fix it. I always had. I had managed our lives so that she was protected and taken care of. I had built a wall around her and the children, healed their cuts and colds and scrapes and bruises. We had always been sure of a storybook ending. Now, for the first time, I was uncertain. I was terribly frightened. The tumor on the monitor was something I had seen in patients who had just months to live. Andrea believed I was a good doctor, and so I was. She believed in my mastery of disease. But we talked less about the patients who couldn't be saved, for whom every treatment I knew and accepted as effective still led inevitably to death. The grim reality had always been a step removed. I had faced cancer as a professional, never as a husband.

I nodded. I'll try, I tried to tell her with a look and a squeeze of her limp hand. We're in this together, and God, how I will try.

She smiled in return. Uncertainly. The full impact of the news had yet to hit her. But amid fear and confusion, she managed to find bravery, and in her sign of bravery I was able to find hope.

W E had to know right away if the cancer had spread. An aide arrived to wheel Andrea, still groggy, from the recovery room to radiology. Doctors Kurtz, Turnbull, and I followed. As stunned as I still felt, I counted as our blessing my job that allowed us such quick access to medical procedures. In the midst of cursing our luck, I knew Andrea and I were fortunate.

Bob first wanted a sonogram. Dr. Jose Botet met us at the door of the room where he would perform the procedure. Different organs and growths produce different sonic echoes. When sound waves are aimed at the body, the echoes that bounce back can be assembled into a picture. A sonogram can identify stones in the gall bladder, kidney stones, and cysts. It can identify blood vessels and show, with computerized coloring techniques, the direction and rate of flow within those blood vessels. It can distinguish new growths on a landscape of healthy tissue, which was what Dr. Botet would be looking for in Andrea.

Botet and Bob discussed the case briefly. Then Bob, Turnbull, and I moved away while Botet oiled Andrea's abdomen to ready her for the procedure. The oil would allow him to guide the sound wave–transmitting probe easily back and forth across her belly in close contact with her skin.

My eyes, and Bob's and Turnbull's, fixed on the monitor as the echoes formed pictures. There was utter silence in the room, a collective holding of breath. The images grew clearer. Starkly, frighteningly clear. I watched in horror as they resolved into spots on Andrea's liver. They were definite, multiple, and widespread.

Dr. Botet shook his head. "I don't believe it," he said. "Her symptoms are too recent. It can't have spread to the liver already. I want to do a CT scan to be sure."

Andrea was wheeled away again. The doctors followed to a control room. I fell in behind them. They were my colleagues, but a separation had occurred. I was the patient's family, to be insulated from the raw bad news. My face felt novocained.

In the room with the CT scanner — it stands for Computerized Tomography, a system that combines x-ray and computer technologies — a nurse positioned Andrea flat on her back on a motorized table. An electric motor hummed, the table moved into a narrow tunnel, she was bombarded by x-rays. Like the sonogram, the CT scan would differentiate between solid and hollow structures, and normal tissues and tumors.

I watched the monitor numbly as the CT scan confirmed the sonogram's results. The cancer had metastasized and was attacking Andrea's liver.

A dull roar filled my head. The smell of my own rank sweat rose to my nostrils, and I struggled to keep breakfast down. I wished insanely that I had never brought her to the hospital, never insisted she be tested, then maybe all this would not be happening. We could wake up and everything would be fine. Before today, Andrea had been to the hospital four times in her life, to deliver our three children and once for a breast biopsy. I remembered the anguish of that biopsy, and the exquisite relief when it turned out benign. Now the sophisticated tests told a different story. I had ordered the same tests many times. I believed them without question, entered their results on patient charts, conveyed their bad news with sympathy and understanding. Now Andrea was the patient, and I was the inconsolable husband quaking on the other side of the doctor's desk. The test results weren't just information, they were a death knell. I couldn't shake the thought that Andrea probably had only months to live, not the long years we looked forward to enjoying.

"Why operate?" Dr. Turnbull turned from the monitor and looked at me, then at Bob. "If the tumor's all over her liver, we're not going to cure her with surgery."

Turnbull, blunt as he was, was simply honest. A metastatic cancer is one that has appeared at a site in the body distant from its original site. When that happens it's usually too late to remove just the original cancer and expect a cure. And a cancer that has reached the liver has reached a virtual greenhouse. All of the digested nutrients absorbed by the intestinal tract are passed into the liver through blood vessels and lymph channels before going elsewhere throughout the body. Whatever is planted there grows very well, including cancer cells. A few isolated spots in the liver might have been cut out. But these were spread throughout, and that was not an option.

I was more concerned about the tumor in Andrea's stomach. It was her choice, not mine, to accept or reject surgery. But I knew if she had any chance to live, it would begin with removal of that tumor. I knew Andrea so well. With an eating disorder already, thinking of the tumor in her stomach would make her stop eating altogether, and she would quickly fade away. Surgery would relieve her fear of the gnawing thing inside her. She was in no shape to make a decision on her own. She still was recovering from the sedation, the invasions and intrusions of the tests, and the shock of the diagnosis. She could not have absorbed what had happened in the last few hours, the pros and cons of the various options, so I did what I was used to doing. I made the choice for her.

"She has to have surgery," I said. "It's the only way she'll have a chance."

Bob supported me. "It's a big tumor," he said. "It could perforate. It's bleeding. She's anemic, she's in pain. It may not cure her, but surgery will be palliative, at the very least."

Turnbull agreed to operate the following Monday.

Chapter

3

"I T's not fair," Andrea cried.

We were in a cab going home. She clenched her fists and beat them on her thighs. "I was planning to finish therapy. I was close. I was ready to live again, and now I'm going to die. It's so fucking not fair." She bit her finger to stifle a sob and turned to stare out the window.

The cab driver caught my eye in the mirror. What are you going to do? he seemed to ask.

"You're not going to die." I took Andrea's fists and uncurled her fingers, held her hands, and tilted her face back to me. Her eyes were wet and troubled. "Don't cry. It sounds bad, but everything's going to be okay. Things will be fine. We'll fight this together. We can do it. We can."

"I have cancer," she said.

"It's cured every day."

Her eyes wanted to believe me. So did I.

Andrea's sense that she was near the end of therapy had encouraged us both. She had struggled to make sense of her childhood and the events there that underlay her anorexia. She was the younger of two daughters. Her family lived in Forest Hills, a New York suburb where the U.S. Open tennis tournament was held before it moved to Flushing

Meadow. Andrea was an active and creative child. That annoyed Andrea's mother for some reason, and she clamped a lid on her expression. Things had to be her mother's way. On her mother's orders, her father nailed Andrea's high chair to the wall to keep her from moving it around. He sawed the rockers off her rocking horse to keep her from rocking. Later, Andrea decided she wanted to be an actor or a dancer. She laid elaborate plans. She attended acting workshops, and applied to New York's High School of Performing Arts, the highly selective *Fame* school. She talked of hiring an agent. Her mother laughed at her. And when she was accepted to the High School of Performing Arts in both dance and drama, a rare accomplishment, her parents refused to let her attend. They wouldn't hear of it. She would meet undesirable people. A traditional high school was safer. Andrea complied with their wishes. On the surface, she did as she was told, but her compliance eroded her. In response to her parents' overwhelming power, she took control of the one area accessible to no one but herself — her body. She asserted her will by depriving her body of nutrition and herself of the pleasure of eating. It was all the worse because Andrea knew food and followed good restaurants and great chefs.

The deep sense of unworthiness touched nearly every aspect of her life. Our relationship, her relationships with the children, the way she related to the world around her, all bore some mark of her childhood. Andrea had struggled to find resolution, but the process had been long and torturous. Now, believing she faced death, she had the doubly bitter sense of being cheated of life.

The cab dropped us at the apartment building. The uniformed doorman pushed the revolving door for us. He started to say something, but changed his mind and smiled politely. Apparently our faces showed how drastically the world had changed.

"What are we going to tell the kids?" she said as the elevator rose to the twelfth floor.

"I don't know." I hadn't thought of it until that moment. I had assumed Andrea would tell them. She was closer to them than I, had been the one who primarily raised them, while I worked.

"You're going to have to tell them," she said.

How? I wondered. How would I tell my sons that their mother might never smile upon their choice of brides, and my daughter that she might lose the chance to know her mother as a friend? I was an immigrant family's first-born son, the hope of generations, the first in my family to graduate from college, a physician whom everyone in the family called when they had a pain. I had always had the answers. Now I felt powerless, as a father and as a physician. How could I admit that I had not protected them?

Andrea, still groggy and slightly nauseated from being sedated, and emotionally drained, went straight to bed. Jonathan was still at work. Joanna would have been home from school, but she didn't seem to be in the apartment and must have been somewhere with her friends. I heard the sound of a television and followed it to Daniel's room.

When he was a baby and still the only child, I had carried Daniel on my back while Andrea and I explored Israel. Later, he had climbed my pants legs to greet me when I came home from work. In time, however, he became a terror, throwing tantrums and refusing to go to school. He was profoundly intelligent, and we didn't understand his behavior. It was disruptive and bizarre. As it continued, occupying center stage and absorbing much of the focus of our family, it eventually led us into therapy.

I stood at the door of his room and he turned to me, his black hair in tight, tousled waves reminding me, as it always did, of Andrea's. He caught my expression and his dark eyes, also like hers, filled with concern. "What?" he said.

"They found a tumor."

"Oh, no. Where is she? Is she okay?"

"She went to bed." I stood there in the doorway and told him in the gentlest words I could find what I thought he should know. But there was no gentle way to say she might have just months to live.

He rose and we held each other. Neither of us could hold back tears. "Don't worry. She'll be okay," he said. "Do Jonathan and Joanna know?"

The phone rang before I could answer him. Picking it up, I heard Joanna asking Andrea, "How did it go?"

"Not real great," Andrea said. "They found a small tumor." But her voice managed to mask her concern.

"Oh. Well, I'm across the street," Joanna said, naming a girlfriend. "I'll be home in a little while."

Joanna was sixteen, intense, and earthily beautiful. Lately it had seemed that I sometimes didn't see her for days at a time. Andrea had told me she had a new boyfriend, and if she wasn't with him, she was with her friends like the girl across the street, young people she had grown up with in our neighborhood.

She arrived home half an hour later. Andrea had gotten up in the meantime. Joanna looked at her sitting at the kitchen table. She looked at me still in my jacket and tie, home at the unusually early hour of four-thirty in the afternoon, and her face clouded.

Andrea rummaged in some lacquered boxes and produced some recent photographs. She said, "Sid, we have these pictures. Why don't you and Joanna go across the street and buy some picture frames?"

Joanna's mouth fell open. It was almost comical. Her expression told how ludicrous it was. It said, "What's going on? She's got a tumor, and they're talking about picture frames?"

But I took the photographs, and Joanna followed me out of the apartment. She began to pepper me with questions before we reached the elevator. Downstairs, I tucked the photographs in my coat pocket and we sat down together in a lounge area in the back of the building's lobby. "How bad is it?" she asked, crying. "Can they take it out? Will she get better?"

I wish I knew, I said. I told her that I thought it would be okay, maintaining the illusion that I could handle it. But she also deserved to know the truth. "It could be really bad," I said. "There's a possibility she could have just a few months."

"A few months? Oh, my God." Joanna jumped up and ran out of the building back to the comfort of her friends.

I sat by myself for a few minutes, feeling unbearably lonely under the weight of my responsibility, just as powerless to soften the blow my daughter felt as I had been unable to protect my wife.

Jonathan, our middle child, was home when I went back upstairs to the apartment. He was sitting in the bedroom with Andrea as she choked out the news that she had a tumor that had spread to the liver. He looked at me, plainly confused, somewhat frightened, wanting to help but not knowing what to do.

He followed me into the living room. "You know what happened today?" he said. "Somebody mentioned Mom was at the hospital for tests, and I joked about it. I said it must be an ulcer, caused by too much stress from her children. It's not a joke, though, is it?"

Once again, I could give no comfort. I said that in most such cases the patient lives no more than a few months. As I spoke I wondered how I could be handling things so badly. It was something I never told my patients and their families. It destroyed all hope, and I don't know why I gave such a harsh prediction to my children. How could I not be gentle with them at such a crucial time? I suppose I said it because I was human; it was what I was thinking, and I blurted my fears because I wanted and needed their comfort. To be able to protect them while I was reeling with shock perhaps was expecting too much of myself.

I tried to protect them in another way, by never saying the word "cancer." All three of them remembered that. I told them that Andrea had a tumor, said that maybe she had just months to live, but I never uttered the word. I never told patients they had cancer until I had seen the proof under the microscope, but there was something else. I couldn't, perhaps for the reason that Susan Sontag highlighted so vividly in *Illness As Metaphor*. Cancer, in our society, meant death. It was the word itself, not the prediction, that conveyed the fatal prognosis. I knew it wasn't necessarily true. I myself had seen many patients cured, but I still could not permit myself to say it.

It also conveyed a sense of failure. I was the father, the head of the family, the provider, healer, and protector. I had this need, this drive, to keep protecting everybody. I was the rock, and I had crumbled. Cancer, the partner in my life's work — that's how it felt, the way one great athlete needs another to push and prod him to great feats — had turned on me and caught me with a sucker punch. Cancer had attacked my wife, despite all I had done to assure my family of a smooth, safe passage through the shoals of life. To acknowledge that Andrea had cancer meant I was no longer in control.

This, too, played into the mythology that had arisen around cancer. The idea that it was some stealthy, malevolent enemy waiting to attack the innocent and unsuspecting formed the basis of my reaction. I felt blame, as if the predator had crept through some gap in my defenses.

That night we gathered around the kitchen table. The table in the dining room was larger, but the kitchen was a kind of family crossroads, where we snacked and caught up with one another. It was the place for morning coffee and late night cocoa, where over the years Andrea had shared the children's pride in their accomplishments, met their friends, and listened as they poured out their troubles and frustrations. Sitting in the kitchen brought us closer. Now we needed each other as never before.

"How can everything change so fast?" Joanna blurted.

Jonathan, her soulmate when they were younger by virtue of our having spent so much time focusing on Daniel's problems, tried to comfort her. But nobody had an answer.

We could have fallen apart then. Our despair could have widened the family fissures until they cracked beyond repair. We were like most families, appearing more ideal than we really were. The stresses on us included the intensity of my work, Andrea's continuing anorexia, and the growing pains of three smart children coming of age in New York City. We thought we had taken a mature and sensible approach to working things out. Therapy would help us keep our balance on the tightrope and lead us slowly to resolution. Until today, we had thought we had all the time in the world.

"It's how things happen," I said. "And nothing's really changed, besides. We're all here around the table. We're a family. We'll stick together, and be brave. We all have to go on doing what we're doing, and work hard, and together we can get through this."

"Do you really believe that?" Andrea said.

"Yes, I do."

"We can remember that we love each other, too," she said fiercely. "I love you, Sid. I love all you kids so much. I can't believe this is happening to us. It makes me mad."

We went on, each of us, to say we loved one another. We had never done it all together, only individually. We felt naked and exposed, and it was hard to find the words. We meant them, though. We all were crying. It was almost as if Andrea were gone already.

The kids dispersed, all trying to handle it in their own way. Jonathan went to a monster truck event at Madison Square Garden, an activity so far from his normal interests it could hardly be imagined.

Later, in bed, Andrea lay rigid, staring at the ceiling, her eyes red from crying. I tried to embrace her but she turned away. "Don't," I whispered. "Let me help you."

"How? How can you help me? How can anybody?"

"I don't know. But let me try. We have to try."

She sighed as if to say it was no use, but she turned back to me and let me hold her. I held her tightly, as if she might float away and my grasp could keep her here on earth, as if by holding her I could keep her next to me forever, and we drifted into troubled sleep.

YOU never think flowers will grow at ground zero. On that first day, and in the days immediately afterward, I said words of reassurance I in no way felt. I believed our lives were over.

I failed to see that Andrea's cancer, of all things, would wake us up. I knew least of all that my beliefs as a doctor were about to be turned upside down.

But I'm going too fast.

That Saturday, five days into the new year, I sat in a book-lined office on 82nd Street off Riverside Drive and cried. I was already sure it was the worst year of my life. Dr. Casper Schmidt sat folded like a praying mantis in a worn, armless leather chair and waited. Schmidt was Andrea's psychoanalyst. Our history with him dated to 1982, when we were trying to fathom Daniel's tantrums. I don't remember now how

Andrea found him in the first place, but when Daniel refused to go with us to his office, for a consultation, Schmidt suggested that she invite him to dinner.

He arrived in a coat and tie. I introduced myself. "Hi, I'm Sid Winawer," I said.

"Hello," he responded. "I'm Dr. Schmidt."

That set the tone of our relationship. That evening, he saw subtle emotional tension between Andrea and me. Andrea, passive on the surface as she had been with her parents, felt anger toward me that she was failing to express. Daniel, with an acute sensitivity to the nuances of our relationship, had become her emotional proxy. His tantrums and stubbornness expressed her anger. Frustration that I felt, over her anorexia and her sitting at home and not working, also was not properly expressed. When Daniel played his role in this triangle, I dismissed him. By dismissing him, I was dismissing her, and he reacted by acting out more. Schmidt explained all this. Daniel displayed the symptoms, but Andrea and I became the patients, learning to express our feelings as they should have been expressed, in order to treat him.

Daniel visited Dr. Schmidt infrequently at first, then regularly. He went alone, with Andrea and me, and to sessions that included all of us. He occupied the center of our family drama. Jonathan saw Schmidt occasionally, Joanna just a few times. My visits to Schmidt had declined over the years, though I still saw him when I had something on my mind, and I sometimes went with Andrea. Only she had felt the need to embark on intense analysis that took her to Schmidt three days a week. With all of this, Schmidt became something of an elder to our family.

Drawing on what I assumed was a Freudian background, he had probed her childhood to find the cause of her anorexia. He placed the blame on her parents for squelching her curiosity and sense of fun and, ultimately, her dreams. Nailing down her high chair and cutting off her rocking horse's rockers were the most vivid, and horrifying, examples of why she had had to take control in the only way she could. I don't know if that was the only reason she wouldn't eat, or couldn't. But she felt she was figuring it out, and that had encouraged both of us. Her cancer took us both back to square one.

Dr. Schmidt was middle-aged, tall, and slender. His short gray hair gave him the stately appearance of a bust on a Roman coin. He moved in the deliberate manner of flamingos feeding. His Dutch-accented speech traced to South-West Africa, now Namibia, where he was born. His medical degree was from the University of Pretoria. He had an impressive knowledge of opera and the classics. The floor-to-ceiling bookshelves in his fourth-floor office were crammed with books on all subjects; books were stacked on the floor beside his chair. Like all Freudians, he spoke little and encouraged his patients to reveal themselves. I sat facing him in a chair that matched his, and just cried my heart out.

Crying came naturally to me. Beautiful violin music, a passage in an opera, a moment in a play, could get me started. I cried when my mother died. I cried when my sister Rita died; I was only four, she was eight, she had an ear infection that progressed to meningitis. In those days before antibiotics, such unchecked infections could eventually penetrate the meninges covering the spinal cord and spread in the spinal fluid to the brain. I didn't know where she had gone, and I could see even then that my father couldn't make sense of it, either, and I cried for both of us. Later, my parents had two other daughters, my sisters Joyce and Hinda, but Rita's death and my father's anguish may have been the force that inspired me to be a doctor. It was a way of controlling the forces that took children from parents, and brown-haired, brown-eyed, freckled sisters from their little brothers. In Schmidt's office, I cried only for myself.

"I don't know, I keep wondering, was it something I might have picked up earlier? I wanted her to have a checkup, but I didn't really push. Were there signs I didn't notice? What can I do now? I want to save her, but I don't know how. I don't know what to do to help her. Help me. Tell me what to do."

Schmidt must have thought we were helpless to decide things on our own. It had become routine for us to use him as a sounding board at times of family crisis, as if we couldn't trust ourselves. We discussed with him many of the important decisions in our lives. He listened, guided us, but moved us to make our own decisions. It was like growing up again and correcting the mistakes.

"This naturally is a terrible thing," he said. "But you have great resources at your disposal. It is within your power to see that she gets the best that medicine has to offer."

I still needed his comfort when I left. I said, "I feel as if I need a hug from you."

The embrace he gave was comforting. I went forth resolved to use all my energy and knowledge, all the medical contacts I had amassed, to help Andrea.

THAT night, Andrea and I went to a movie with the kids. We saw *Hamlet,* the Franco Zeffirelli version with Mel Gibson. Why we sought diversion from our own unfolding family tragedy in one of the great tragedies of all time remains a mystery to me. Why not a comedy? In *Hamlet, everybody* dies. I suppose the darkness fit our mood. Andrea closed her eyes and went to sleep with her head on my shoulder. Hamlet met his fate because he could not make up his mind. I resolved anew not to let Andrea suffer from indecisiveness. In the dim light of the theater, I repledged my unconditional support.

Chapter

4

ANDREA grew nervous as Monday's surgery approached. On Sunday, I drove her across town to Dr. Schmidt's office. She went on her own during the week, but if she scheduled an extra weekend session, I often drove her. This was an emergency appointment prior to the operation. She drummed her fingers on the car door and flipped down the visor to check her makeup in the mirror as we crossed Central Park at the 85th Street transverse.

I dropped her off and found a parking space. I usually enjoyed this hour by myself, to have a cup of coffee and a warm bagel while I read the *New York Times*. This time, the coffee and the bagel cooled while I waited in deep thought, trying to adjust to the idea that Andrea was going in for major surgery. Some of her agitation had rubbed off on me. Sometime later, her knock on the window woke me from my trance.

"What happened?" Her composure as she got into the car stood in stark contrast to her earlier distress.

"Sid, I've decided not to have surgery tomorrow. I need to build my strength up. A few days in the hospital with some good nutrition, and then I'll go ahead." She clicked her seat belt into place and smoothed her coat.

"Was this Dr. Schmidt's idea?"

"Yes."

"I didn't know he knew anything about nutrition." I couldn't keep the edge from my voice. Where did Schmidt get off dictating a surgical schedule?

"Stop it, Sid. He knows a lot. He said it's one of the things I need to do to beat this thing."

"Shouldn't your doctors decide that?" I was shocked by her sudden resolve, and angry with Schmidt. My colleagues had plenty of experience and good judgment. They knew what was best for her. What had Schmidt put into her head? I knew he had pursued another medical specialty, gynecology, before taking up psychiatry. From what I saw in his office, he read the medical journals. But he wasn't an expert in nutrition, internal medicine, or cancer, and advising her to postpone the operation struck me as interfering with her care.

"No," she said, in a tone that dismissed further discussion. "I'm the patient. I should decide."

I was in conflict as we drove home. I didn't think Schmidt's advice made sense. It opposed medical opinions I respected. Besides, I had argued for her surgery. Postponing the operation would be against my medical judgment. I agreed with my colleagues. At the same time, I wanted to back her and support her. I faced for the first time the dilemma I would face again and again: doctor versus lover, the choice between medical knowledge and unswerving support. I knew Andrea placed great trust in Schmidt. She had a pilgrim's faith in the mind's powers and in psychotherapy's potential. Schmidt was her guru. He had helped us with Daniel, and in her view he had helped our family. His word had the effect of holy writ. In the psychological process of transference, she probably saw him as a father figure. So I could support her, moving away from what I knew to be medical truth, or let her argue for the postponement on her own.

"Sid, you won't make me have the operation tomorrow, will you?" she said as we were pulling into the garage at the apartment building.

I couldn't let her fight alone. I turned to her and said, "I told you we were in this together. I'll help you."

Late that afternoon, she packed toiletries and clothing. She packed oversized T-shirts to avoid wearing the hospital gowns. I had told her how shapeless and anonymous they made her look. She also packed a Walkman tape player and a tape Dr. Schmidt had given her. I knew the music — Isaac Stern on violin and Yo-Yo Ma on cello playing the Brahms Double Concerto. The composition was Brahms's last orchestral piece, composed with two musician friends in mind. It endured as a metaphor for two lives in tune, lived closely. It exuded hope and seemed to calm and exalt the spirit all at once. If the beauty of a work of art could provide a reason for living, this Brahms concerto did so.

Brahms. Dictating the schedule of her surgery. I didn't see the connection then. But over the next weeks and months, it would appear to me with the force of revelation. Much about Casper Schmidt disturbed me. Andrea sometimes seemed to be a puppet in his hands. But his intentions were good. In introducing her to the seemingly opposing concepts of serenity and self-empowerment, he was helping Andrea begin to understand how to use her mind against her cancer.

ANDREA was calm. I was like Woody Allen's character in *Take the Money and Run,* fretting over whether he should wear his blue suit or his brown suit to rob a bank. How should I get her to the hospital? I obsessed. Should I call a cab? Should I take the car?

Finally I stopped and asked myself, What the hell difference does it make? I asked the doorman on duty to hail a cab. Then the kids decided to go with us, and I took the car instead.

We entered the hospital this time through the main entrance. As we sat in the waiting room, I experienced again that sense of disorientation from being on the other side. Andrea had her little bag beside her, like an orphaned child being sent to an aunt's. I held her hand. Around us, others sat waiting their turns. Faces were serious, nobody talked much. They were probably thinking, as I was, of their lives before the diagnosis. Scenes from our honeymoon, from Daniel's birth, from Jonathan's and Joanna's, flashed in my mind's eye and disappeared. Everything known and certain was in the past. The future waited behind closed doors beyond the waiting room. I knew the anxiety I felt must be shared by every patient's family.

"Winawer. Winawer." I looked around for a phone to see who was paging me. Then I remembered I was not being paged for a consultation. We were next in line.

In a small room, an admission clerk asked questions and entered our answers into a computer. He copied my insurance card. Andrea officially became a patient.

She was still unpacking in her room when her parents arrived with her sister, Marsha, and Marsha's husband, Bruce. Helen and Michael Bloom had retired from Forest Hills to Florida fifteen years earlier. They were staying with Marsha and Bruce in New Jersey. Helen was flame-haired and normally formidable, still dictating everything that went on around her. My preoccupation with Andrea didn't prevent me from seeing that Helen looked drawn and ill. As if to apologize for the change in her behavior, she complained of being tired. She was seventy-four, Michael eighty-seven, and she had kept her husband on a short leash as long as I had known them. Helen gave the orders, and Michael found it easier to comply than to argue. On his own, he was generous and easygoing, and Andrea truly loved him.

Whatever Andrea's history with her parents, she needed them now. She held her mother in a long embrace, as if to emphasize her gratitude for her attention.

Then Joyce, my sister from Long Island, burst into the room. Joyce, a mental health administrator, was a fountain of enthusiasm and affection. She smothered everyone, but especially the children, with hugs.

Andrea and I were alone later when Bob Kurtz and Alan Turnbull arrived. Turnbull started to brief her about tomorrow's surgery, but she interrupted him. "Alan, I'm sorry, but I just can't have surgery tomorrow. You're going to have to postpone it. Dr. Schmidt says I'm too weak. I need some nutritional buildup, then I can go ahead."

"Who is Dr. Schmidt?" Turnbull asked.

"He's my psychotherapist." And I do everything he says, she might have added.

Dr. Turnbull looked at her, then at me, and then huddled in the hall with Bob. Andrea was five-five and weighed about 102 pounds. They both thought she was thin and underweight but strong enough to undergo the operation.

"What do you think, Sid?" Bob asked.

I thought she could use some extra pounds, but that was nothing new. As Chief of Gastroenterology, I was also Chief of Sloan-Kettering's Nutrition Service, and I knew a few days of nutritional supplements could not possibly make a difference. That was my view as a doctor. But I wasn't her doctor, I was the patient's spouse, and I had told her I would help her. I took a breath and said, "It's up to her. If she feels the need for extra nutrition, she should get it."

They both looked at me. I felt like a traitor to what I knew was good medicine. I felt nervous that they'd think I had suddenly become a crackpot and was not to be trusted. I could hear the whispers, "Poor Sid," and I resented Schmidt's interference all the more. But the die was cast, and there was no going back. My way lay with Andrea.

They argued with her, but I wouldn't join them, and she could not be moved. Dr. Turnbull rescheduled her operation for Thursday.

"I WON," she said. The other doctors had gone, and all the relatives were back at our apartment with the kids. We were alone in her room. There was surprise in her voice, and pride. It erased my misgivings. I was glad I had supported her.

"You sound surprised," I said.

"I am, a little. But I know it will help. Dr. Schmidt says I'm in for a long fight, and I have to be ready. I have to be strong."

I tried to remember when I'd seen this kind of determination before in Andrea. Certainly she had devoted herself to things she cared about. She had been determined to marry me, determined in pregnancy, labor, and delivery, determined in creating the environments in which we lived. But this was different. She swam with the current on those occasions. Now she was swimming upstream against strong, authoritarian opposition, bucking the current in a way she had never done against her parents. I wondered if it would continue and how I would react if it did.

Early Monday, a ray of hope arrived. Bob had taken biopsy tissue during the endoscopy, and it produced an unusual and surprising pathology report. Andrea's cancer turned out not to be the usual type of gastric cancer, but a carcinoid tumor. Carcinoids can arise anywhere in the body, including the stomach. They occur in nests of cells — neuroendocrine cells — that release hormones in response to stimulation from the nervous system.

Sitting in the hospital cafeteria over coffee, I spilled out my excitement to one of my close friends. Dr. Moshe Shike was Memorial Sloan-Kettering's Director of Clinical Nutrition, but he knew the implications of tumor types as well. Most carcinoids are indolent. They are stable or progress slowly. Patients can live more or less normal lifespans of twenty years or more. Some are aggressive, but those are more likely than gastric cancer to respond to chemotherapy.

"My God, Moshe, I thought she was going to die in six months," I said, choking up. "Maybe now we've got a chance."

Moshe waited until I could speak again. He smiled, showing the same gentleness and consideration I knew he displayed with patients. "That's good news," he said. "So it's even more important to get her that nutrition that she needs."

I could have hugged him for that. Come to think of it, I did, there in the cafeteria with technicians and nurses and doctors in green and white coats looking on. It was Moshe's way of showing that a doctor could support a patient even when that patient resisted a medical consensus.

He placed Andrea on a high-calorie diet with supplemental formulas. The diet and supplements he prescribed added calories in the form of protein, fat, and carbohydrates. Andrea got vitamins and minerals that she needed.

She showed no signs of anorexia in the next few days. She needed no intravenous feeding. Able to get her calories in solid food, she attacked her meals with a gusto I had not seen in years. She ate large portions of a variety of foods — chicken, fish, and starches in the form of pasta — and I could almost see her mental computer adding up the calories. It was as if she had willed her anorexia away.

By Wednesday night, when she had to stop eating so she could receive anesthesia the next morning, she had gained more than two pounds. Two pounds for Andrea was monumental.

"Two pounds, Sid," she said proudly. "I feel good about the operation now. If I come through it, I think I'll be able to handle whatever happens next."

"Don't worry, you'll come through it."

But she knew she could die on the operating table. It was a slim, but realistic, possibility. She wanted all the children to come to her that night. She spoke to each one privately, making sure nothing was unsaid.

Joanna told me later what her mother said: "Joanna, if you were to fall in love, and the boy wasn't Jewish, you know, that would be all right. If you wanted to live with him before you got married, that would be all right. If you wanted to weave baskets in New Mexico, that would be all right, too. If you were to think about that, and think about asking me, if I weren't here, that's what I would say. You just have to live the way you feel is right for you."

I cried when I heard that. It was wonderfully generous. She had poured herself into the children, and the hardest thing a parent has to do is let them go. Andrea really wasn't ready. She wanted the children to keep needing her. But now, she was giving Joanna permission to fly without her, if it came to that, and I'm sure she did the same with Daniel and Jonathan.

WE all were nervous the next morning. We moved silently about the apartment as we got ready for school and work. Shirley arrived to do the housekeeping, and went about her tasks with a troubled look. Joanna left for school thinking, she told me later, "My mother's going under the knife."

I rushed to the hospital and Andrea's room in time to give her a kiss and a hug. Attendants helped her from the bed onto a stretcher and wheeled her away down the hall. My last image was of her lying on the stretcher with earphones on, listening to the tape of the Brahms Double Concerto as she received sedation. She was smiling.

I retreated to my office to wait. Soon Jonathan came in, neglecting his temporary job. Marsha appeared, having driven from New Jersey. Moshe Shike came in and took a seat. Bob Kurtz stuck his head in the door to say he was heading for the operating room and would be back later. My very close friend Don Lefft was there. Others entered, saw the group, and added to it, dragging chairs from other offices to pull up around the conference table. We talked tensely about how the surgery was likely to turn out and what it might mean for Andrea's survival. After a while there was nothing to say, and the conversation drifted to school, family, work, anything to distract us. My eyes kept finding, on the shelves lined with books and journals that testified to my career, the family photographs. We were at the beach, skiing, celebrating one another's birthdays. Our smiles seemed so innocent and unsuspecting.

My thoughts weren't on the conversation. I prayed that Alan Turnbull would not find Andrea's abdomen full of cancer. If the tumor was too widespread, he would not be able to resect — a word whose Latin root means "to cut off" — the tumor from the stomach. The plan in such surgery is to remove the cancer with some surrounding normal tissue so as not to leave any tumor present, but retain enough of the stomach to allow it to accept a decent-sized meal. The entire stomach can be removed if need be. A person can survive without a stomach, even without an intestinal tract, if intravenous nutrition is provided. But that's a last resort, and nutrition and weight loss problems can occur, especially in a thin person. If the cancer is too widespread, it may be impossible to resect a portion of the stomach. There is nothing to do then but close the incision and leave things as they are — an "open and close" operation. Today, fortunately, advanced preoperative assessments made possible by CT scans and other tests have made these cases rare.

By late morning, we were running out of conversation. Each pause grew heavier with tension. Suddenly, the door swung open and Bob flew into the office. Our heads all turned on cue.

"It went well," he said. "The tumor in the stomach was localized. Turnbull got it all out, and she's in recovery."

We all breathed again.

Bad news followed the good. It wasn't unsuspected. Dr. Turnbull had taken tissue from the spots on Andrea's liver for a "frozen section" — a quick fix of the tissue so it could be examined immediately. The spots were indeed cancerous. The frozen section results were preliminary. They would have to be confirmed by standard pathology procedures. I had hoped the spots somehow were benign, but it was a faint hope, and now it slipped away.

I rushed to the recovery room. When Andrea opened her eyes I was standing there holding her hand. She was still woozy and could hardly speak, but she croaked out one question over and over. "Did he take it out? Did he take it out?"

How glad and relieved I was that I could say, "Yes. Yes," over and over as I shed tears of crazy relief. Surgery clearly had been the right decision. We had conquered today. We could worry about tomorrow, tomorrow.

At home that night, an insistent reggae beat sounded from Joanna's room. I listened at her door. The singer was Bob Marley, who died of cancer in 1981 when he was only thirty-six. Joanna was singing with him. Every little thing, they sang, was going to be all right.

ANDREA'S parents returned to Ft. Lauderdale following the operation. She recuperated in the hospital for several days. My workday provided frequent breaks when I could see her, but the evenings were free and uninterrupted. The kids came in according to their schedules, but mostly it was just the two of us. I appropriated the floor's VCR cart and we watched old movies.

Old movies were a passion of ours, and *Dark Victory* was a favorite. Bette Davis plays an heiress with a brain tumor; surgery saves her, and she and her surgeon fall in love and embark on a glorious romance. It turns out that the surgery is effective only for a year, but what a year they have. *A Star Is Born* was another, in which Judy Garland's rising star remains faithful to her husband's memory. Love and death were our preoccupations.

The final pathology report confirmed that the spots on her liver were malignant. This I expected, but still more bad news followed. Surgical removal of the tumor, the surrounding portion of the stomach wall, and adjacent lymph nodes permitted a far more comprehensive picture of Andrea's cancer than did the endoscopic biopsy, based on a relatively small tissue sample, and the "frozen section." The story the larger tissue sample told was revealed under a microscope.

Steve Sternberg reviewed the slides with me. Another excellent member of the Sloan-Kettering staff, Steve is one of the leading authorities on surgical pathology and the author of a widely used textbook in the field. He bent his head to one set of eyepieces on a multiheaded microscope while I looked in the other. The cells we looked at came from the stomach wall, the blood vessels that traverse the stomach, and the surrounding lymph nodes. They all showed the dark blotches and irregular edges that indicate cancer. Cancer is really a group of about 150 different diseases that can arise anywhere within the body. All cancers, however, share one important characteristic — uncontrolled cell growth. Cancerous cells have no respect for borders. Their invasion of healthy tissues looks like an ordered field of wheat being devoured by a swarm of locusts.

Steve's eyes met mine over the eyepieces of the microscope. He didn't have to say a word.

The report confirmed that Andrea's tumor was a carcinoid. I clung stubbornly to the hope that it was indolent.

That hope, too, was dashed. "It's an atypical carcinoid," Steve said. These neuroendocrine carcinomas, as they also are called, occur less frequently than the indolent type, and usually behave quite differently. In most cases they are aggressive, spreading early and rapidly. Rarely, they behave like the indolent types and are less aggressive.

I prayed this was the case with Andrea's. It was just a prayer. We were not going to win on the diagnosis. We had only one path to follow. She needed to regain her strength quickly. She would need every ounce of strength to fight the cancer, whatever its course was going to be.

Chapter

5

ANDREA was in the hospital for eleven days. We had not been separated at night for that long since our wedding.

Classes resumed at Columbia, and Jonathan returned to his dormitory at the uptown campus. Daniel decided he would not return to college in New Hampshire. "I think I should be here," he said. I helped him find a job at Sloan-Kettering. Joanna resumed life as a teenager, which meant school, friends, and as little time at home as possible. They were concerned about Andrea, and me, and did their best to be supportive. But they were no substitute for Andrea's presence and companionship. I missed her. I missed the sound of her voice and her laughter, her warmth and the feel of her in the bed beside me, I missed closing my eyes knowing she was there and waking up beside her in the morning. Alone late at night in the bedroom scented with her presence, I found myself remembering.

We met in 1967. I was a confident young doctor with a position I had always wanted. My return to New York the year before, from Boston and a Harvard faculty position, was a triumphal homecoming for a boy from Brooklyn whose parents had struggled. We had moved from one neighborhood to another as my father worked to support my mother, me, and my sisters. I attended public school and yeshiva in Brooklyn, graduated from New York University, and returned to Brooklyn for medical school at Downstate Medical Center, part of the state university system, where I could afford the low tuition.

Medical school at first was hard. During two years of lectures and lab study, I fought to remember that each step took me closer to realizing my boyhood dream of joining the exalted ranks of doctors. But as soon as I entered the hospital wards for my clinical clerkships, I knew I had found my place. The wards were alive with challenges and mysteries in the form of patients needing care. I would stay up half the night trying to unravel them, even on my nights off. I read charts, poured over texts in the library, and sought the company of "real doctors" in the cafeteria.

To make money, I joined a group of students who covered the clinical lab at night at Long Island College Hospital, one of Downstate's affiliated hospitals. The salary was $100 a month plus room and board. Cash, food, even the dormlike quarters at the hospital, were a windfall I embraced ecstatically. Between that and my summer job as a bellhop in the Catskills, I could pay my way and contribute a little to my parents. One of my proudest moments was earning enough one summer to carpet the living and dining rooms of their apartment. I worked right through my internship and residency in Internal Medicine at Maimonides Hospital and the Veterans Administration Hospital in Brooklyn. By then my medical education was advanced enough to get a job working as a ship's doctor on the last great U.S. ocean liner, the S.S. *United States,* during my vacations. This was a dream. I wore a uniform with gold stripes, white or navy blue depending on whether the ship was cruising the Caribbean or crossing the Atlantic. Women vied for a spot at my table in the dining room. I treated seasick passengers, and staved off seasickness myself by maintaining a slight buzz at the open bar in the evenings. After my residency, I spent two years in the Air Force as a captain in the Medical Corps, stationed at Langley Air Force Base, Virginia. Then, I began thinking of a specialty.

Gastroenterology attracted me. It was a newly blossoming field. Emerging technology such as the endoscope allowed doctors to see into internal organs, examine their appearance, and study their structure and function. Much of the new work was being done in Boston, and I landed a two-year fellowship with the Harvard Medical Division at Boston City Hospital. When the fellowship ended, I stayed on for two additional years as an instructor.

It was a formative time. I taught, treated patients, and conducted research. I loved it all: late nights in the lab or on the wards; the sleuthing that the new instruments permitted; intervening to diagnose and change the course of a disease; discussions with my colleagues. We spoke our own language. Our knowledge was special, our power enormous. We had the sense that we were pushing back the frontiers of medicine.

I fell in with Dr. Norman Zamcheck. Chunky, slightly bald, hard of hearing, Zamcheck was a creative thinker. I found in his company both mental stimulation and something of a father figure. "Z" was a big talker. New ideas made his eyes light up. He would entertain any possibility. We talked for hours about medicine and life, free-associating from one idea to the next. He believed in conventional medicine, proven in rigorous research. But conventional methods, he said, were conventional only until something replaced them. Typical of most researchers, he pushed the envelope to gain new knowledge and insights. He encouraged an openness to therapies and thoughts outside the mainstream and taught me that research was the exploration of new vistas and unproven beliefs.

I dated a lot in those days, but never felt like settling down. One girl, when I was in medical school, forced me to choose between her and the books, and I had to choose the books. In Boston, I asked a girl to marry me, but she turned me down. "You're going to be an academic doctor," she told me with an accountant's eye on my future. "You're not going to make enough money."

An academic doctor doesn't have to live in poverty. But the practice I had in mind did include teaching and research along with seeing patients. And I wanted to see them at a hospital, not a private office. Such positions were available. I bided my time and began to present the results of my research at medical and scientific meetings of groups like the Boston GI Society and the Eastern Gut Club. The Gut Club was a group of academic GIs — gastrointestinal specialists, as gastroenterologists were also known — from schools like Harvard, Boston University, Johns Hopkins, and Columbia. We got together twice a year. People got to know me, and with the emergence of the new era of gastroenterology, I started getting offers.

All the while, I had continued to visit New York. I came primarily to see my parents and my sisters, but the city exerted a pull of its own. I missed its museums, concerts, the opera, its overall vitality. And now I could afford it all. I was a nice Jewish boy, a doctor, a "catch," and New York was full of bright, accomplished women. I kept thinking about what a ball I would have back in New York, professionally, culturally, and socially.

Then came a great opportunity. The Cornell Medical School offered me a teaching position that included appointments at all three Cornell-affiliated hospitals in New York City — Bellevue's Cornell Division, New York Hospital, and Memorial Sloan-Kettering.

I left Boston and a cramped studio apartment for the excitement of my "hometown." It was 1966. I was driving a green Pontiac convertible. My new apartment, in a just-completed high-rise at 86th Street and Second Avenue, was big and the building had a swimming pool. A lot of young people were moving in. Yorkville, the surrounding neighborhood, rang with the accents of Germans and eastern Europeans who had lived there for years. People came from all over the city to their restaurants. At newsstands and fruit stalls and shops, the area vibrated with life.

At first I was headquartered at Bellevue. I treated patients, taught, spent long hours in research, and wrote papers and grants. After a few months my main headquarters moved from Bellevue to Memorial Sloan-Kettering. There, my interests turned to gastrointestinal cancer and cancer prevention. I played as hard as I worked, dating to the opera, to concerts and plays, to movies and restaurants. I took a summer share in a beach house in the Hamptons and a share in a Vermont ski house in the winter. I even had time to use the pool at the apartment building. I was quite the bon vivant young doctor.

I had stopped thinking about marriage after I was turned down in Boston. But I soon found, returning to my big, new apartment after making some interesting scientific observation, that the excitement of discovery fell flat when there was no one to share it with. The apartment felt empty. I felt empty, too.

The winter after I returned to New York, a friend of mine arranged a blind date. He and his girlfriend invited me to dinner at their apartment with a student at Columbia who was studying for her master's in audiology.

I almost skipped it. I was coming from the unveiling of my grandmother's headstone at a cemetery on Long Island, a gloomy prelude to a date. But the minute I met Andrea Bloom, I was glad I came.

FIRST impressions. That Audrey Hepburn face, of course, right out of *Breakfast at Tiffany's*. She was twenty-two, but she had so much more presence than I expected in someone her age. Her body language was eloquent, her movements filled with grace. She was slender, her hair glossy black, like ebony, worn in a swirl. Her smile was warm and inviting. When her dark brown eyes met mine, I felt that our souls had touched.

Was it love at first sight? It was years later that one of her college roommates wrote me that Andrea's song was "I'll Know (When My Love Comes Along)" from *Guys and Dolls*. We certainly were drawn to each other across the Brooklyn–Forest Hills divide. I was thrilled by her interest in the arts, her love of music, her passion for drama and ballet. Audiology wasn't something she cared about, she said; her parents pushed her into it. Teaching deaf students was safer and more secure than the stage career she would have loved. She had attended Boston University during the same four years I was at Boston City Hospital, and we laughed at the coincidence of that. Another of her roommates was a premed student, and they had often eaten together at the hospital cafeteria. We passed unnoticed by each other then.

After dinner, we danced. It was really more like rhythmic swaying in each other's arms; my friend's tiny apartment had no room to dance. We danced to ballads of young love, mostly by the Beatles. She held on tight, even when the music ended. I felt special and loved in her embrace.

We slept together that night in my apartment. In the morning, I asked her to tell me her last name again, and she laughed and punched me on the arm. It wasn't as casual as it sounds. It was the Age of Aquarius, but I don't think we were reckless, or selfish, just having sex for the sake of sex. We connected from the moment we met, and we made love as the first expression of a romance that we both sensed from the start.

We were together every weekend from then on. I enjoyed the space she gave me during the week, but as Friday neared I looked forward to her coming, and on Friday night when I got home I couldn't wait for the call from the doorman, saying with a wink in his voice, "Andrea is here." She loved the apartment; it was everything her Columbia dormitory room was not — it had food in the refrigerator, plenty of room, and was on a high floor far from prying eyes at other windows. We would make love and walk around nude; order Chinese food and eat sitting on the floor with candles and a bottle of wine; idle away mornings curled up on the sofa with coffee and the paper, Andrea wearing only one of my shirts, looking so wonderful my heart turned inside out.

She was always moving. She swayed back and forth waiting for the elevator, and she loved rocking chairs. It was only later that I learned how her love of movement had been squelched when she was young.

The first time I took her to the opera, we saw *Madame Butterfly* at the Met. She wore a short tight dress, and as we strolled around at intermission I felt the eyes of other couples on us, making me feel proud to be with such a beautiful woman.

My feelings toward her grew stronger with each passing day and week. She worked hard to encourage them. Andrea made me feel she understood me and appreciated the excitement I found in my work. She perceived my need for a partner, someone with whom I could share companionship, love, warmth, and intimacy. It was as if she could see inside me. I had found my soulmate.

She dropped hints, but I still resisted marriage, for some reason. "You're too young for me," I said.

When she replied, "In what way am I too young?" I had no answer.

Then one night the phone rang. It was a Sunday at the beginning of December 1968. A bachelor friend of mine was calling to say he and his girlfriend had decided to get married. Andrea heard my end of the conversation and sensed that I was weakening. "Let's do it," she said when I hung up the phone. "Let's get married. What are you afraid of, Sid?"

An hour later we were in my car, driving through a blinding rainstorm on our way to Maryland.

We crossed the state line and checked into a motel. Andrea insisted that we sleep in separate beds. The next morning, Monday, December 2, we got our blood tests and a marriage license. Then we found a justice of the peace. He read us the marriage vows and declared us man and wife. We walked out of his office and I turned to her and said, "What about a couple of kids?"

She always used that to remind me that I had been ready, after all.

Our wedding feast was lunch at the Occidental Restaurant in Washington, D.C. The waiter who served us liked the fact that we were newlyweds. He entertained us with his jokes and took a photograph. We were seated against the wall under pictures of Capitol Hill celebrities. Andrea was wearing a baby blue suit and a fuzzy white hat shaped like a shako; I wore a navy blue blazer, and in those days had sideburns. I still have the check from that meal. With wine it cost $17.27, plus the tip. After our banquet, we drove back to New York.

Our families took it pretty well. They of course were happy we were married. Eloping was a different story. My parents had themselves eloped, but Andrea's father wanted a real wedding for his "Annie." He had a clothing store in Far Rockaway, and with her mother looming in the background, he put his salesmanship to work.

"We don't want you to do anything you don't want to do," he said to us. "But consider this: It's a special time. If you'd like to have a little ceremony, a wedding, I'd be happy to help you do it. Only if you want it. But it might be nice. Annie, if you walked down the aisle, if you had a white dress on, your mother and I would be so proud. But only if you want it. But as time passes, a couple of years from now, you may look back and wish you had a wedding to remember. Just think about it."

He was the velvet glove, her mother was the fist. Her nickname for Andrea was Cookie. "Have a real wedding. You'll break your father's heart, Cookie, if you don't. You'll regret it as long as you live."

When we agreed, her father turned his persuasion to the details. "How many people do you want to have? I know you want to keep it small. But think about your friends. No more than a hundred . . ."

So we were married again, by my childhood rabbi this time, at the end of December at the Bayswater Jewish Center in Far Rockaway. The religious ceremony, shared with our families and friends, seemed to cement the marriage. Since we had a real wedding, we had to have a real honeymoon. We flew to Nassau, where we spent New Year's Eve. One night at Paradise Island, Andrea played roulette. She couldn't lose. A crowd gathered and started cheering for her. Other women were rubbing their money on her to get a dose of her luck. I watched her and saw that she loved it, loved the hands reaching out to her, the adulation, the validation in such contrast to her parents' dismissal of her dreams when she was a child. I knew she would always be the center of my life; I would always validate and appreciate her.

I thought her winning was a sign of things to come for us, the beginning of our lucky streak.

We felt like two kids on the threshold of life. We were going to have a family and have a great time. We were going to enjoy ourselves, have fun with each other, soak up what the city had to offer, play the game of life. The future stretched on forever. That's the way it is for lovers starting out. We didn't feel like we were grown up. We really never did.

We always thought there would be time for that.

I BROUGHT her home from the hospital on January 17. A week after her surgery, Andrea still had a little pain, but she felt strong and in good spirits. She felt good, in retrospect, about insisting on the postponement of her surgery. She thought that had helped her sail through the operation and it seemed to have made her more optimistic.

The building's doormen lit up in smiles to see her back again. Shirley greeted us at the door of the apartment, ignored me, and drew Andrea into an embrace as she asked, "Andrea, how are you feeling, girl?" Then she released her like something hot, afraid she'd hugged too hard. A few minutes later, Andrea was in bed and Shirley was taking her hot soup.

Home was a happy change from the hospital environment. Our bedroom was everything the hospital was not. Andrea had created an environment that was cozy, warm, and sexy, a haven from the world. We would retreat here in the evenings, turn off the phones, and crawl into the king-size bed among the Ralph Lauren patterns and soft colors and lighting, the plentiful big pillows, to read, talk, make love. It was a citadel where nothing could harm us. For Andrea now, it meant home. Normalcy. Safety. At least for a while.

Home was only a temporary respite. With the primary tumor removed, Andrea's doctors focused on the next phase of treatment. They weren't sure what was best. They knew she had a neuroendocrine cancer that had spread. They thought it was aggressive, but so far could not be sure. Was it aggressive or, less likely, indolent? Should they hit her with really strong chemotherapy, with all its side effects, immediately? Or should they observe the enemy for a short time to confirm its biological behavior before embarking on a long and strenuous course of treatment?

"Let's wait a month," Bob Kurtz said finally. "Then we'll take a new CT scan to see if the cancer has progressed."

"Wait?" Andrea was incensed. "How am I supposed to wait? I want to do something. What if it has progressed? I'll be a month behind."

"I understand. But it's important to do the right thing. And to not do the wrong thing," he added.

A month. Four weeks. Thirty days, more or less. I listened to Bob and heard myself telling patients to postpone the knowledge of their fate. I thought of all the times I had said to patients, "I'll see you in a month. We'll repeat the test."

"I'm not going to be able to stand it," Andrea said on the way home. "I'm going to have to figure out something to do. I don't know what, but something."

The month loomed like an eternity. Hours would inch by. Days would crawl like glaciers. Like Andrea, I couldn't stand the idea of a month of inactivity while, perhaps, the cancer gained. I wondered how patients and their families stood this waiting game.

It was at this point that I think it hit home to me that I was a cancer patient's spouse. Earlier, I had acted like a doctor, and I still felt the impulse to dictate a course of treatment. Now, Andrea was frustrated. I was, too, because there seemed to be nothing I could do. I recognized in myself men and women I had seen in my office. They wanted information, resolution. Most of all they wanted action. They wanted to help but weren't sure how as their loved ones faced the painful mysteries of cancer and its treatment.

Now I was one of them. I had never realized how isolated from the process many of them felt. Their pain did not show up on their loved one's sonogram or CT scan. An endoscopy did not reveal it. The pain was assumed, even acknowledged, but it was rarely addressed. I couldn't remember recruiting many spouses to join their loved one's fight. As a doctor, I had tried to be supportive. I had tried to be warm and understanding and to offer hope, but Bob had been all of that and more, and now it seemed not to be enough.

Andrea and I both needed to do more than wait to be told what to do next. I needed direction, skills, some starting point to see how I could help Andrea effectively. By effectively, I mean that I needed to participate in her struggle, not as a doctor would by directing treatment, but finding a partnership with her that made me more than just a sympathetic observer. Andrea, too, needed a point of preparation. She had made a good start by dictating the schedule of her surgery and by sticking to her new diet. Now she felt the need to do more.

I was looking at cancer from a different perspective for the first time.

Chapter

6

T H E frustration of waiting prompted me to call Casper Schmidt for an appointment. He asked me to bring a copy of Andrea's pathology report. He read it while we sat in his book-filled consulting room. The sounds of traffic on Riverside Drive filtered through the window. At last he raised his head from the report describing rampant cancer cells that had spread into lymph nodes and the blood vessels of the stomach wall and to the liver. "Has she seen this?" he asked.

"No," I told him. "We've discussed it, but she hasn't actually read it."

Bob had given her the essence. I had gone a little deeper, sketching its conclusions in layperson's terms. Pathology reports are crammed with hard-to-grasp, potentially frightening medical terminology. I didn't know any doctor who made a practice of showing them to patients.

"She deserves to know the details, don't you think?" he asked in his crisp accent.

"It's not necessary. No doctor would do it with a patient. It would be very unusual."

I had specific reasons for keeping the full report with its harsh details from Andrea. I was trying to protect her; I didn't want her horrified. No one but a therapist would be prepared to deal with the outpouring of emotions the clinical details could produce. Schmidt, I suspected, had the audacity to do just that.

Andrea had an appointment with him the next day. It was a Sunday, and I dropped her off and went for my coffee and bagel. After the allotted fifty minutes, the door to his building flew open and Andrea ran down the steps. She threw herself into the car, crying as she slammed the door behind her. I knew instantly.

"He showed you the pathology report."

She nodded, sniffling.

I cursed Schmidt in my heart for his arrogance and cruelty. I was right, seeing the report had devastated her. Its medical language was a clear and bleak portrait of life-threatening cancer. I had no doubt Schmidt had given her a full translation. He had told Andrea that the cancer, in invading her lymphatic system, was poised to spread throughout her body. It seemed to me that this was tantamount to taunting a lynching victim with a picture of the gallows. He had rubbed her nose in her sickness and tormented her with the probability that she would die. I questioned his ethics in showing her the report without asking me and in interposing himself in her treatment.

She retreated into herself on the way home, held herself together in the elevator. Once in the apartment, she fled into our bedroom and shut the door. She had read her own death sentence. I could think of no words to console her, so I left her alone.

An hour later, she emerged. I looked up from the newspaper, groping for comforting words, but I stopped when I saw that her eyes were clear and her jaw set.

"He's right," she said. She continued before I could reply, sweeping her arms in a dramatic flourish. "What if I were ignorant, Sid? What if I didn't know? If I thought that with the tumor taken out, the spots on my liver just would dry up and go away, how stupid would that be? Dr. Schmidt's right, I can't deceive myself. I can't afford to believe things are better than they are. I have to know what I'm fighting here. This is life and death. If I know the enemy is strong, I know I have to be strong, too."

I looked at her. More probably, I stared. She was animated, bristling with determination. I wondered what Schmidt knew that I didn't. He was able to raise my wife to new powers of resolve. Had he been right after all?

His giving her the full picture was very difficult for me to accept. And even if I had been convinced at the time that it was the thing to do, I don't think I could have done it. It would have been emotionally impossible. My instinct to protect her was too strong. I thought it would destroy her hope and send her into a depression. This was a good example of why a doctor should never treat a loved one.

I had underestimated Andrea. I had always known, as a doctor, that my patients divided themselves into two groups: those who help themselves and those who don't. The patients who knew and accepted that the stakes were high were more prepared to fight. For some reason it surprised me to learn that Andrea was in that group. I never imagined that she was capable of absorbing that pathology report and using it to empower herself. But in not protecting her, Schmidt was demanding that she grow, and she was responding. The harsh portrait of her illness had mobilized rather than depressed her. I resented Schmidt not only for being right, for having the courage and wisdom to do what I could not, but also for being more in touch with my wife's psyche and hidden capabilities than I was.

I wasn't sure I knew the Andrea I saw emerging. I thought I liked what I saw, but I wasn't sure of that, either. She frightened me a little. If Andrea was gaining strength and power, I had more than ever to find some similar resource. I had some way to go in my new role as the patient's spouse.

We both, in those days, were at the beginning of a journey. Andrea's struggle was destined to draw us closer, show us new priorities, and bring improvement beyond measure to our lives. But I did not yet fully understand and embrace what I had to do, which was to support in every way her self-empowerment.

I took my first steps by cutting back on my practice. I reduced and reassigned my usual clinical, administrative, and research activities. I stopped giving lectures and canceled my trips to local and national medical meetings. I resigned from my temple's board and stepped down as chair of the social action committee whose activities included running a soup kitchen and arranging home visits to the elderly. These things were important, but others could take the reins now. Andrea needed my full attention. I felt the need to not let anything slip by. How much had been slipping by all these years? I wondered. How much had I missed?

As I was making these decisions, Andrea kept moving forward on her own.

"This cancer is a cosmic kick in the ass," she declared one morning at the kitchen table. A bowl of steaming oatmeal sat in front of her. She had been eating well, had grown stronger, her pain was reduced to tenderness, and she was tired of staying in the apartment. "I feel like there should be a cosmic way I can kick back."

When I got home that evening, she was reading one of Dr. Bernie Siegel's meditation books.

Andrea was an armchair student of psychology. She had always been fascinated with the mind's capabilities, its resilience, and its enormous untapped powers. This fascination grew out of her experience with psychotherapy and also her deep regard for Dr. Schmidt. Intelligence in a person was the quality she admired most. She had done quite a bit of reading on the subject. Soon after her surgery, when she was still in the hospital, she had asked a staff psychiatrist for something new to read, but nothing was available. She was frustrated, because she needed first to cope with the stress that all cancer patients have. Then she wanted to know how to apply the powers of her mind toward better health and, if possible, to use it to help her body rid itself of cancer.

I had never taken Dr. Siegel seriously. Trained as a surgeon, he began exploring meditation and other techniques and gave up his surgical practice to become a leading advocate of mind-body healing. His books and tapes were (and remain) phenomenally popular, and I, like many conventional doctors, viewed him with suspicion. I suspected him of leading bewildered people into unproven areas while they rejected treatments that could help them. Let me apologize.

Conventional medicine can be insulating. I was a conventionally trained gastroenterologist and oncologist working in the world's foremost cancer center, surrounded by colleagues similarly trained, with the same conventional perspective. Under normal circumstances, our clinical interactions are constant and intense. We talk about patients every day, hold weekly conferences in each department, meet frequently on a center-wide basis, all to keep our knowledge, clinical skills, and approaches up-to-date in conventional terms. That is not to say we don't seek new approaches. Being an academic center, we constantly develop new protocols and try new drugs and new and better diagnostic methods. Sloan-Kettering for years had studied the stresses and anxieties that affect patients with cancer. However, the bottom line of that research — that patients do better if they receive a range of self-empowering psychological supports — had not entered the day-to-day thinking of most physicians. I certainly had not woven it into the fabric of my practice.

The millions who flocked to Siegel's work apparently had done so because he gave them something they found lacking in conventional medicine. He gave them more hope and directions on how to help themselves. He wrote about patients with death warrants, like Andrea's, who decided, "To hell with everybody, I am going to survive, or at least I will enjoy to the fullest the time I have remaining." And in the cases he related, they did just that. They survived by helping themselves — they demanded to know the course of treatment, they added components of their own, and ultimately they forged a strong belief in their ability to guide their destiny.

And if they didn't survive, their lives at least were improved for the time they had left.

Were these miracles, spontaneous cures, that Siegel described? I don't know. But I was beginning to understand that patients facing lethal diseases have to find hope, and the start of hope is the belief that they can help themselves. Help themselves to survive, if that is possible. At the very least, help themselves to live well and die by their own rules, not those of the disease.

Andrea needed a consistent source of hope. So did I. First, however, she needed to find a way to take her mind off the cancer. Siegel suggested a meditation technique called guided visualization, a way of displacing fear of the disease with beautiful thoughts.

The first time Andrea meditated on a place of beauty, I only watched. Skeptically. She closed her eyes. After a moment or two, her breathing deepened. The pinch between her eyebrows and the set of her mouth slowly eased like ripples vanishing from the surface of a pond. As the tension left her expression, a slight smile appeared. She continued breathing with a deep and steady rhythm. She seemed calmer and more peaceful, but I wasn't sure if what I was seeing was real. I thought maybe she was aping the effects of meditation to impress me.

She opened her eyes after a few minutes. She blinked, as if waking after sleep. She saw me watching, and flashed a smile that seemed warmer and less brittle. "Well, that was nice," she said. "You should try it."

Afterward, not only did she speak with a tone that suggested hope and optimism, but her movements and gestures, even her walk, were more relaxed.

Seeking an explanation for these changes, I recalled medical school lessons about the way the mind controls the body's functions. The brain asserts direct neurological control over the basic activities. For example, you don't have to think about it for your heart to beat, your lungs to breathe, or your intestinal tract to digest food. Beyond that, but short of the level of thought-directed activity, a critical point in the mind-body relationship lies at the juncture of the brain and the pituitary gland.

The pituitary sits at the base of the brain and is the master gland of the body. Neurons of the brain in close proximity to the pituitary secrete molecules called peptides. These have a profound influence; they control the pituitary's hormone secretions, which in turn control the hormones released by all the body's other glands, including the adrenal and thyroid glands, and the ovaries and testes.

These hormones — triggered by the pituitary — feed back to the pituitary in a marvelously sophisticated, self-correcting system that shuts off when the pituitary senses they have reached the right levels.

The key word is balance. In a healthy body, the hormone levels are balanced to allow the glands and the body to function properly. But this looping feedback system can be affected and set off balance by a number of factors, including stress, nutritional status, and illness.

Certain rhythms also affect the ebb and flow of hormones, in ways that most people feel but don't really recognize why. The most obvious, the female menstrual cycle, follows a more or less monthly rhythmic pattern. Hormones also rise and fall in a twenty-four-hour cycle. An even shorter rhythm occurs every five to ten minutes.

Researchers for years have attempted to decipher these rhythms. Anticancer drugs applied in synchronization with the twenty-four-hour circadian rhythm seem to maximize their tumor-killing effect. Cancer is not the only disease that seems to ebb and flow in some relation to the body's rhythms or the rhythms of the universe. Ulcers, for example, have an intrinsic periodicity that makes them recur commonly in the spring and fall. Fever tends to rise higher in the evening.

We have much to learn about these rhythms. We do know that they are controlled through the brain and its influence on the pituitary gland, and in turn through the effect of the pituitary on the other glands of the body. We know that they can be upset by many things. Depression, stress, poor nutrition, too much alcohol, certain drugs, and certain diseases all tip the body's rhythms out of balance.

The word *balance* returned again and again as I thought of the seemingly profound effects of meditation on Andrea. The calm it brought on was obvious. Andrea was stressed by the threatening diagnosis and uncertainty of waiting for a course of treatment. The meditation restored her surface equilibrium, and I could only think that beneath the surface it was restoring her body's rhythms to a state of balance. In a healthy person the balance of rhythms would help maintain good health. It stood to reason it would help Andrea regain it.

IN that month of waiting, Andrea embraced meditation wholly. It was her escape from thinking of the cancer. Bernie Siegel's visualizations led her to places that were free of disease.

She kept asking me to meditate with her, but I resisted. It seemed nice for her, but was not something I thought I needed. Eventually, I sat with her to humor her and went through the motions. I mostly fell asleep.

But Andrea had a way of plunging into something new that was contagious. She began to meditate four and five times a day. Each time the cancer tapped her on the shoulder and said, "Think of me," she sat quietly, closed her eyes, and found a refuge. As I saw how good it was for her, my resistance weakened.

Andrea had always liked my voice. I used to read poetry to her when we were dating, and she loved it when I read from Shakespeare's *Sonnets*. We got out of the habit after we got married and the children came along. Now she wanted me to read aloud from Siegel's book. I felt faintly foolish, but I agreed, and we sat side by side on the bed, holding hands.

Following Siegel's imagery, we followed a path along a bridge over a slow-moving river to a spot among lush trees, where we felt a soft breeze and the sun on our skin, heard birds sing, and smelled the flowers that grew in profusion along the riverbank. Looking up from the page, I saw that it gave Andrea such comfort and I felt we were indeed in this beautiful place together. We had found a focus other than the cancer — a Shangri-la of the mind. I was not just her expediter, reading while she listened. I was her traveling companion, too. I felt a surge of togetherness with her that was almost overwhelming. To be with her was the most important thing, and we had made a new journey together.

Once the ice was broken, I began reading to her every night.

I told myself for a while I was doing it only for Andrea's benefit. Then I realized that I, too, was feeling its effects. I became calmer as I read to her and we entered the new place. I relaxed as I watched her relax, felt her hand gripping mine slowly lose its tension, saw her face soften into a faint smile. We both forgot our fear and found safety in gardens of the mind. The visual meditations relieved us of tension and made it possible to sleep.

Chapter

7

I N early February, at the end of our month of waiting, Bob Kurtz slipped the x-ray film from the new CT scan onto the view box and stepped back. I looked, and quickly turned away.

"God, Bob, look at it," I said when I got over my sick feeling.

Andrea's liver was being consumed. It looked like Swiss cheese, with many more spots, and the prior spots had grown frighteningly large. This was not a stable cancer. We were dealing with an aggressive neuroendocrine carcinoma that was growing rapidly, following the deadly and relentless course we had feared.

"It doesn't look good, Sid," Bob said sympathetically. "But remember, it's a type that's highly responsive to chemotherapy. Almost everyone who has this goes into remission. There's a protocol reported by the Mayo Clinic you and Andrea should look at."

He described a new chemotherapy protocol appropriate for small-cell carcinoma of the lung, which was the model for Andrea's cancer. It combined the powerful chemical agents cisplatin and VP-16.

"They've done a clinical study and have seen some excellent responses," Bob said. "I think she should get started on this right away."

My emotional reaction was to resist the chemical invasion of Andrea's body. Chemotherapy is usually used to treat cancer that has spread beyond its starting point, or to prevent a recurrence when the probability of that is high. Physicians use radiation therapy for some forms of cancer to control local growth, among them cancers that have just invaded the adjacent lymph nodes but have not spread to distant sites. Radiation can also control some types of distant spread, cancer in the bones and brain being two examples. A combination of radiation and chemotherapy sometimes is used as well.

I knew chemotherapy alone was the appropriate option for Andrea's type and stage of cancer. It was what I would have recommended. I also knew it was rough. Like radiation, it would attack and kill her normal as well as her cancer cells. It would deplete her so badly that she could take treatment only intermittently, with time out in between the cycles to allow the healthy cells to renew themselves. The cells in her bone marrow that produce white and red blood cells and platelets were the most important. Lack of red cells causes anemia, and platelets are important in clotting to prevent bleeding. These can be replaced temporarily in an emergency, but white cells must regenerate. They are the keys to the body's immune resistance; without them, she would be open to infections that could drive her out of her mind with pain before they killed her.

There was no guarantee, for all that, that chemotherapy would be successful. Maybe the spots of tumor in her liver would grow despite the treatment. They could shrink, but not disappear — a partial response. The best we could expect was a complete response, in which the tumor could no longer be detected.

Bob had said the Mayo Clinic treatment was likely to produce a complete response.

But a total or complete response, despite what the words imply, is often not a cure. Chemotherapy may not eliminate every single cancer cell. Some cells may resist the particular chemical agent that is used. If Andrea's tumor responded, we could not assume it was gone just because it diminished and couldn't be detected. It might only be invisible to imaging techniques. The resistant cancer cells could remain in microscopic clusters, continuing to multiply until they were again visible to scans and detectable by blood tests.

Experience shows that then the chemical agents that worked the first time probably would not produce the same good effect again. The surviving cancer cells would be more resistant. Having survived the initial chemotherapy, they could have developed new survival skills as they lay undetected. In that case they would be harder to wipe out than before and in all likelihood would continue to multiply relentlessly.

A patient is considered cured only with time. Patients who have a complete response are followed for months and then years. Only then, if they have no recurrence of the tumor, are they finally said to be cured. But "cure" is a term used more by laypeople. Physicians prefer to consider that a patient is in prolonged remission. Certain cancers, like breast cancer, can produce recurrences many years later.

However, with very aggressive cancers like Andrea's neuroendocrine type, or lung cancer, the absence of a recurrence in two or three years could indicate a long-term remission or cure.

"The first strike is all-important, Andrea," Bob said as we sat together in his office. He did not show her the frightening image on the slide. He stressed cancer's tenacity and its ability to develop new forms of resistance to a previously effective drug. "The first go-round, you want to go in with all guns blazing. The Mayo Clinic protocol is a good protocol. The chemo is strong, and the trial results are good. It's going to give you some time. I told Sid, I think you should get started on it right away."

Andrea was calm. I was sure she had spent the morning meditating. She nodded thoughtfully and said, "Give me a couple of days to think it over, Bob. Maybe there are some other possibilities."

RETURNING to my office after Andrea went home, I called Sloan-Kettering's medical library. Soon, an abstract of the Mayo Clinic trial results arrived on my desk. I looked it over with the knowledge that here, again, we had an advantage over other cancer-stricken families.

That night Andrea and I ate Chinese takeout with Daniel and Joanna. As soon as we had read our fortunes and cleared away the cartons and the dishes, Andrea and I moved into the living room to study the trial results.

Andrea was elegant even in sweat pants and a big T-shirt. She curled her feet under her and patted the couch, and her Yorkshire terrier, Daisy, jumped up and nestled beside her. Daisy was tiny, a wisp of a dog, a hummingbird of canines.

The room's south-facing windows gave a view down the east side of Manhattan. The objects around us spoke of the comfortable life in which, until a few short weeks ago, we had been cozily ensconced: a big, thick Oriental rug, abstract art by modern masters, a black grand piano that had been silent since Andrea abruptly and without warning stopped her six-hour daily practices. Books on meditation, by Bernie Siegel and the psychologist Dr. Lawrence LeShan, had begun to take up space on the big coffee table. This was to become our war room.

The abstract of a cancer trial is crammed with statistical and methodological shorthand. There's a lot of information contained in its abbreviations, as long as you have the key. I sat next to Andrea and guided her through it. The results were sobering. Patients had an average remission of eight months and an average survival time of fourteen months. The majority of patients had only a partial response. Even those patients with a complete response showed signs of recurrent tumor several months later. The ultimate mortality rate was 100 percent. No one was cured and survived.

She looked up with a puzzled expression. "How can anybody be enthusiastic about that?"

"You're right," I said. "But it's our best shot. What else can we do?"

"I don't know. Something. There must be something."

I looked at the months offered by the protocol, and I agreed with her. We wanted more. More time, more life. "I'll start looking," I said. "I'll run a search."

The next day and in the days to come, I used every resource at my disposal. The years I had spent organizing, studying, and lecturing at national and international meetings on gastrointestinal cancer came into play, and I felt fortunate to have a set of worldwide contacts who, without fail, responded to my calls. I spent hours on the phone with physicians and research scientists, trying to track down the newest data. I spoke at length with Dr. Charles Moertel, the oncologist who directed the Mayo Clinic protocol, and Dr. David Johnson, who as head of oncology at Vanderbilt University Hospital in Nashville had run a similar study with the same results. I ordered computer searches from the medical library, downloaded abstracts of every human and animal study that showed any promise whatsoever. I tracked down pharmaceutical industry researchers for what they could tell me about new drugs still in the testing phases. I was a medical Sherlock Holmes. No clue was too small or too obscure to study as I sorted through the grab bag of possibilities.

I reported to Andrea at the end of each day. She hung on every word. Each search came down to the same answer: no drug therapy was effective for long. There were a lot of brilliant ideas, a host of promising drugs. But nothing had proven it could beat her cancer.

Andrea didn't want theories and promises. She wanted help, and I was desperate to help her find it.

"HAVE you heard of hyperthermia?"

We were — where else? — in Dr. Schmidt's consulting room. A new stack of books and medical journals had risen beside his chair since my last visit.

The psychiatrist had become a part of Andrea's treatment decision making. Whether he was thrusting himself into the picture, or we were telegraphing a need for direction, was not altogether clear. I resented it, but she trusted him and considered his views critical. Since her diagnosis, Schmidt had revealed himself as up-to-date on all manner of current cancer treatments. He seemed to know everything that was happening on the frontiers, whether accepted by the medical establishment or not. I saw no obvious reason for his uncanny knowledge, but he had impressed me before with all he knew about music, literature, and art, as well as medicine. Hyperthermia, however, was beyond esoteric.

Andrea looked at me from her seat on the couch against the wall.

"Well, yes, I've heard of hyperthermia. It's not in the forefront of any cancer treatment that I know about."

Most people have heard of *hypo*thermia — the potentially fatal chilling that unprotected swimmers suffer in cold water, for example. Hyperthermia is just the opposite. A controlled heating of the body to a high fever level, it began as an attempt to stimulate the body's immune system. The concept had been around for years; its history was part of every doctor's education.

The use of high fever in treating tumors was first suggested in 1866, when a physician in Germany named Busch reported the regression of a tumor in a middle-aged woman who had suffered a high fever produced by an infection. In 1891, Dr. William B. Coley, a surgeon at Memorial Hospital in New York City, deliberately produced fever-causing infections in twelve patients with malignant tumors and reported that eight of them responded. Later, he developed a heat-killed vaccine, which became known as "Coley's Toxin." Other scientists found it hard to duplicate Coley's positive results using this early, crude product, and there were side effects, but Coley's pioneering work opened the door to a new concept of cancer treatment. His preparation worked through the immune response that attacked cancer cells, and it was thought that the high fever was part of the process. He was the first investigator in the United States to use this approach to fight cancer. Coley's Toxin produced fevers up to about 104 degrees Fahrenheit, and later research showed it also induced immunological factors, including interferon and other cytokines that are now administered to some patients as part of cancer therapy. As a medical student I had heard arguments that cancer cells were more sensitive than normal tissues are to heat.

In the few recent cases I knew about where hyperthermia was used against cancer, it usually had been on only one limb or region of the body. Chemotherapy had been a component of these treatments. I re-

called that chemotherapy and hyperthermia in combination sometimes produced responses where chemotherapy alone did not. The
heat in these cases was not used to stimulate the immune system, but
to enhance the effect of chemotherapeutic drugs on cancer cells. Extra-
corporeal hyperthermia, in which the blood was heated outside the patient's body, also had been used to treat AIDS, with controversial
results.

"You might look into it," said Schmidt. "I think you should. Call Dr.
Ian Robins in Madison, Wisconsin. He's at the University of Wisconsin's
Comprehensive Cancer Center there. Here, I've got his number."

He said that Robins was conducting trials in hyperthermia and that
his whole-body hyperthermia system was the best, safest, and most effective in the country. How Schmidt knew this, I had no idea. Once
again, I found his intelligence uncanny.

"WILL you, Sid?" Andrea asked as we drove across Central Park on the
way home. The trees in their wintery bareness looked brittle enough to
crack and splinter.

I hated the notion that I was being Schmidt's water boy, carrying
news to Andrea of every crazy treatment he suggested. But she wanted
to know, and I had pledged to use my contacts to investigate every possibility. Besides, I reluctantly admitted that hyperthermia had shown
enough promise to warrant making a few inquiries.

The first descriptions of whole-body hyperthermia I found made it
sound like medieval torture. Patients had been immersed in molten
wax, encased in heating blankets and insulating fabrics, or sheathed in
high-flow, warm water perfusion suits. The intense heat strained their
hearts, kidneys, and brains. Nausea, vomiting, diarrhea, confusion,
seizures, strokes, heart attacks, and irregular heartbeats were among the
reported side effects. Some patients were burned, and some died.

I'm not putting Andrea through this, I told myself. I'd rather see her
in the dungeon of a Transylvanian castle than subjected to such a bizarre
form of treatment. The goal of conventional cancer treatment is not to

kill cancer cells at any cost, but to maintain a good quality of life for the patient. Some toxic drugs, for example, may have such a remote chance of producing good results and such awful side effects that it is better to withhold them.

For all of its macabre aspects, however, hyperthermia still looked intriguing. The most recent reports said it inhibited DNA repair, and thereby lessened the cancer cells' usual resistance to chemotherapeutic drugs.

I kept asking questions and sending out feelers. The M. D. Anderson Tumor Institute in Texas was using hyperthermia, but considered it risky. I could find no other experienced whole-body hyperthermia team anywhere except the one Schmidt had pointed us toward.

As Schmidt had said, the program at Wisconsin-Madison was considered safer than the rest. Dr. Robins had devised a radiant heat chamber that eliminated direct contact with the patient's body. The heat-induced stresses on the body were the same, but there was no danger from burning. Robins was treating patients with hyperthermia combined with chemotherapy. The drug he used was similar to the one the Mayo Clinic protocol was using, but Robins's lab work suggested that the hyperthermia increased its effectiveness by a factor of three to four. It was as if his patients were getting that much more chemotherapy. Such a dose would be difficult for the body to endure if administered directly; it would have disastrous effects on the bone marrow, for example. But Dr. Robins's wife, Dr. Floriane d'Oliere, had discovered, when they were working together in his laboratory, that a side effect of whole-body hyperthermia was its inducement of the growth factors called cytokines, which protect the bone marrow.

Robins's work was sponsored and supported by the National Cancer Institute and the University of Wisconsin. His treatment protocols had passed the university's review board. This was no fly-by-night program. Robins was serious, conducting clinical trials with all the appropriate documentation. The research scientist in me warmed to hyperthermia. I was receptive to pushing out the borders of knowledge.

But a research scientist needs some evidence to move ahead. All the studies on hyperthermia in treating cancer were preliminary. It had never been proved to cure cancer or even prolong life, only that it might cause shrinkage of the tumor. I called Dr. Robins. He told me he had never treated a neuroendocrine cancer like Andrea's.

At the end, I still didn't know what she should do. Mayo Clinic protocol or hyperthermia? I had gathered data obsessively and succeeded only in increasing my dilemma. Andrea and I poured over the statistics night after night in the living room. They bounced back and forth in my brain, but gave me no clear answer. I felt I was literally going crazy.

I swallowed my resentment and asked Dr. Schmidt what he thought we should do. He laced his long fingers together and said gravely, "All I can say is that hyperthermia is something to consider. Whether to use it or not is up to you."

My colleagues at Sloan-Kettering were against it. Bob Kurtz and Dr. Ephraim Casper, Andrea's medical oncologist whom everyone called Fry, urged us to start the Mayo Clinic treatment. Their voices were a chorus, at home and around the world. Dr. Vince DeVita, then Sloan-Kettering's Physician-in-Chief who had come to us from heading the National Cancer Institute, spoke for the overwhelming majority when he told me one day in his office:

"Keep Andrea here and begin the Mayo Clinic protocol. You know how important it is to use the most powerful drugs first."

But the trial results kept haunting me. I and everybody who recommended the Mayo Clinic treatment knew what the statistics said. The most powerful drugs, used first, would keep Andrea alive only for a time. It angered me to think that the chorus urging us to the Mayo Clinic protocol did not believe she could be cured or somehow get a prolonged remission. They were condemning her to a few months. They were willing to accept that she would die in a short time.

I could not accept that. Not long ago I had been a physician who reviewed patients' charts with all the expertise that conventional medicine could offer, and when I saw the obvious was willing to accept the inevitability of fatal outcomes. I acknowledged when the battle was lost. It was important, medically, to know when to stop fighting. But for Andrea, it was much too soon. I was wholly on the patients' side of the equation now. I would not accept it. I refused.

At the same time, I was furious with Schmidt for planting in Andrea's head, and in mine, the idea of this outlandish new treatment with its enormous risks and no proven benefit.

Soon, I found myself in the office of Sloan-Kettering's president and CEO, Dr. Paul Marks. I sat down and told him of my dilemma.

"I don't know either, Sid," he told me. "All I can tell you is that I'll support whatever you decide."

I was grateful for his wisdom. He understood our need for hopeful options and to make an unpressured decision.

The next person I spoke with was Dr. Zvi Fuchs, chair of Sloan-Kettering's Radiation Oncology Department. I stopped him in the corridor and poured out my dilemma. Dr. Fuchs understood, too. "You know what you have at the Mayo Clinic, and it's not good enough," he said. "In Wisconsin, you don't know what you have, but you have at least the possibility of a miracle."

After all that, I still didn't know what to do. I felt all the time that it was my decision. I was not Andrea's doctor, but I felt I was still her medical advisor. I was still the expert, right? I had drifted back over the line between physician and spouse. I was trying to make a doctor's decision, but my love for Andrea had frozen my decision-making capabilities. Wanting so badly to make the right decision and finding no clear path, I couldn't make any decision at all. The emotions were too powerful, the fear of consequence too great. I loved her too much to take a chance on making a fatal mistake.

Chapter

8

I was no closer to a decision after several days. We both felt the urgency of time rushing past. Andrea and I put the dishes in the dishwasher after supper and headed to the living room to dissect the statistics once again.

She arranged herself on the couch. Daisy jumped up and curled into a ball beside her. Andrea stroked the little dog as she arranged her words. Then she took my hand and said, "Sid, I know you've been trying to decide the right thing to do. But it's really my decision. Whichever treatment it is, I'm the one who has to go through it. Nobody else, just me. Right?"

"That's right."

"Well, I've thought about it, and I've decided I want to try hyperthermia."

"Have you really thought about it? Are you sure?" I asked.

"You better know it, Sid," she said with sudden fierce conviction. "One way I buy a few months and ride off into the sunset. The other way, who knows? I think it's worth the chance. Don't you?"

Relief swept over me, and I hugged her tightly. She had taken the decision out of my hands. I also felt a little dread. I would support her without question, but we were going down an unknown path with no guarantees. This could be our only shot. We might be burning our bridges behind us by rejecting the Mayo Clinic protocol. The Andrea who was willing to spin the roulette wheel still surprised me. But as she continued to assert herself in the fight against her cancer, I was starting to get used to it. My surprise was changing fast to admiration.

Not that there wasn't ample reason for admiration in the past. She had, after all, tended to me for almost twenty-five years, borne and raised three children, and spearheaded the construction of a new beach house to replace the one our family had outgrown. She was no shrinking violet. But like many doctors, I tended to assume ultimate control. And certainly, when it came to medicine, she always had conceded. In the prelude to her diagnosis, she had been told what to do, and she did it: "Andrea, go in for a checkup. Andrea, you're going to have an endoscopy. Andrea, now you need a sonogram. Andrea, stick out your arm for the IV. Andrea, let's schedule you for surgery." Until she postponed her surgery, like most patients she was guided totally by authoritative doctors.

But she was right. She was the one who had cancer. Her life was the one on the line. So what if she had chosen the less-traveled road? She was acting with strength, character, and courage, and I would follow and defend her.

The new Andrea was becoming the kind of patient Bernie Siegel writes about. She was energized, empowered, bent on knowing the options and then choosing her own way. Physicians of the old school often are uncomfortable with such patients. They do it all wrong, this new breed. They won't sit idly by and let the doctor make the decisions. They insist on getting involved. They ask questions, and demand answers. They want to take the reins and participate actively in their own healing.

Growing numbers of doctors view patients like these positively.

They are their own best allies, after all. I had seen, and still do in my practice, that such patients are always the ones who help themselves. They are more prepared to fight in the first place because they know the stakes. Then, if they have a treatment plan they believe in, they participate more enthusiastically.

Now that I was on the patient side, allied with an inquiring, enthusiastic patient, I saw even more clearly the importance of a treatment plan negotiated between the patient and the doctor. The doctor-patient relationship should not be a one-way street. Andrea was taking responsibility for her own recovery by choosing a plan she believed in. She had a greater stake in the outcome and was more likely to do the things she needed to do to get well.

Hyperthermia remained an uncertain choice. But I shared her conviction that uncertain hope was better than hopeless certainty. Now we had something to look forward to.

ANDREA told Bob Kurtz that she had chosen hyperthermia over the Mayo Clinic protocol. He understood that we were going for the miracle and this time didn't try to change her mind.

Now we had to persuade Ian Robins to accept her. Bob called him to refer her and discuss the case, but there were several barriers. The first we already knew about: the fact that Robins had never treated Andrea's type of cancer. Beyond that, the doctor in Wisconsin was wary, and I couldn't blame him.

The medical world, like all professions, has its own networks and grapevines. I knew from talking with Robins that he had heard of me and knew my reputation. It is unusual for someone known in the field of cancer treatment to leave his own institution for treatment at another. The same goes for the doctor's spouse.

I knew he probably was thinking, "Good God, Sid Winawer's wife. If I treat her and she dies, there goes my program."

He told me later he was thinking something very much like that. "I wasn't too eager, since it was the wife of a prominent service chief at Sloan-Kettering," he said. "I thought, 'If something goes wrong, it will literally travel around the world.' That was not something I coveted."

He wanted us to act on really well informed consent. He told Bob, "I want them to know what they're getting into."

Bob told us Robins was reluctant. "Call him," he said. "Maybe you can put his fears to rest."

We called him from home that night. Andrea drove the conversation. She had a sense of humor and a wicked, throaty laugh, and she applied them both to her advantage. "Never mind Sid and his many publications and the fact that he's lectured all over the world," she said to Dr. Robins with a laugh. "I'm just another patient."

We held our breath, and then he laughed, too, breaking the tension. He was glad to hear that neither of us expected VIP treatment and agreed to consider her for the program.

To be accepted, she had to pass a battery of tests. Robins emphasized the stresses hyperthermia places on the body. "It's literally like running a marathon," he said. "My patients need the stamina of long-distance runners to endure the strain the high temperature imposes." Andrea would need to run a gamut of x-rays, another CT scan, a brain scan, certain blood tests, and a cardiac stress test.

She was eager to get started. Now that she had decided on hyperthermia, the clock had started running again. In reality, it had never stopped, but she again felt the cancer gaining. Robins administered the hyperthermia treatments only twice a week, and he had a waiting list. Each day took on new importance. Bob did his part, taking Robins's list of tests and administering them all within three days.

One produced a potential roadblock. The electrocardiogram during her stress test showed inverted "T" waves. This potentially damaging anomaly is a signal of possible ischemia, a circulation problem around the heart caused by coronary artery disease. The cardiologist who read the test thought it was an electrical variant and within the normal range. Robins was not convinced. I was learning that he was a meticulous physician with a suspicious streak. He would look at a potential problem ten different ways before proceeding.

The waiting, again, was the hardest part. Andrea was desperate to start treatment. I was desperate to help her. "Look, let us propose a compromise," I argued on the telephone while she listened nervously on an extension. All I wanted was to get him to open the door enough so we could stick our feet in. "Let us come out there. We'll bring all the test results, x-rays, scans, and cardiograms. You can give her another stress test. We'll accept your judgment about the results, whatever it is. If she passes, she'd like to begin the treatments right away."

Robins agreed, and we made plans to fly to Madison, Wisconsin.

THE waiting didn't get any easier. The uncertainty filled us with anxiety and made the few additional days stretch out like weeks. Andrea and I, Daniel and Joanna, and Jonathan, who shuttled back and forth from Columbia, each occupied his or her own separate bubble of preoccupation. Nobody put it into words, but we all felt that we were approaching an unknown place where anything could happen, a place like the blank spaces on ancient maps, where legends warned explorers, "There be dragons here."

Daniel felt this most of all, perhaps. He remained sensitive to Andrea's moods and feelings. As Schmidt had identified early on, he took on her fear and pain as if it were his own, as her "empath." Now, as on the day of her first tests, he mirrored her agitation. Joanna retreated to her boyfriend and her books to escape the tension. Jonathan called from his dormitory and asked to use the car. He had made his own plans for escape, with a weekend ski trip to Vermont.

The children were Andrea's proudest accomplishments. We attended Lamaze natural childbirth classes together. I coached her through each labor and delivery. She bore each child naturally, delivering it into the world on the "crest of labor pains," as she would say. Waves of the ocean were her metaphor, the pain not engulfing her but lifting her and carrying her on to the next crest. After each crest she would smile with the joy of having ridden the wave that much closer to the safe shore of delivery. She breast-fed each baby. Pictures I took of her, swollen with milk and so very young, as she fed Daniel, still evoked tender feelings in me. Still later, she nurtured them through kindergarten, school, and music lessons.

We were scheduled to leave on a Sunday. The Friday before, Jonathan arrived to pick up the car for his ski trip. He got as far as the Triborough Bridge and rear-ended another car at a tollbooth. He surprised us by showing up back at the apartment, shaken, to say a tow truck was bringing the car home.

"Driving was the last thing on my mind," he said. "I was thinking about Mommy."

"Don't worry about it," I told him. "It's not important as long as no one was hurt." Dr. Schmidt told him later that he was responding subconsciously to his mother's wish that he stay home. By far the quieter of the two brothers, Jonathan's emotions were not on display as Daniel's were.

Andrea paced Saturday away. Daniel followed her around, telling jokes to try to make her laugh. Sometimes, they laughed together at my expense, joshing me for being too serious, the doctor in the white coat. These were metaphorical pokes in the belly, Daniel said. Today, the jokes fell flat. Andrea found it hard to laugh. She disappeared periodically into the bedroom, where I knew she was trying to meditate in private. Joanna disappeared, but called now and then to ask, "How's Mommy doing? Is she okay?" She and Andrea were close in the way that two women have to be in a family where the men outnumber them.

Andrea and I left for LaGuardia Airport on Sunday afternoon. We were happy to be moving at last.

The waiting was over. No matter what happened, action was better than doing nothing while the enemy advanced. That was the spouse talking, eager to help Andrea get on with her plan.

The physician, boarding the plane, felt rising anxiety. I had forgotten, until I squeezed into an airplane seat among strangers who wore baseball caps and spoke in the big, hearty tones of the Midwest, just how much I was a creature of my institution and hometown. I depended on my colleagues at Sloan-Kettering, on the familiar collegiality of medicine, on my friends and my extended family, on the supportive atmosphere that we were now abandoning. The plane took off and I wasn't sure anymore. My commitment to help Andrea was just as strong, but my medical doubts returned. I thought of questions I had forgotten to ask. The dangers of hyperthermia loomed larger, while the potential benefits diminished in my mind. The faith I had in Robins slipped a little.

But as we flew farther west and neared our destination, Andrea slept and the spouse-physician struggle gave way to a kind of psychic exhaustion. I was tired of fighting within myself. The physician yielded, for the time being, to the spouse. Andrea had made her decision, and I backed it. The die was cast, and we were on our way.

W E reached Madison after changing planes in Milwaukee. It was cold, a deep Wisconsin winter cold. We rode a cab from the airport that took us along an ice-crusted lake through snow-covered fields. Snow lined the city streets and smoke rose from chimneys. Lights were blinking on as twilight fell.

Robins had given us the name of an inn near the hospital. Weirdly, people were walking around the lobby in shorts, as if after being outside they wanted to shed the weight of winter clothes. Andrea said she thought Midwesterners must be really hardy people.

The next morning, a taxi dropped us at the door of the University of Wisconsin Hospital and Clinics. It was a sprawling stone-and-glass building, and its big, open lobby greeted us with the familiar sight of men and women in white coats and mint green scrubs, hurrying. We waited while a receptionist paged Dr. Robins.

"Here he is now," she said after a few minutes.

A man with mussed black hair, prominent cheekbones, and an outdoor squint approached across the lobby. "Ian Robins. Welcome to Madison," he said.

Robins's posture and manner exuded confidence. Though not tall, he was commanding: powerfully built under his white coat, he intruded into the space ahead of him the way a fighter might crowd an opponent. Later, I would learn that he had black belts in judo, jujitsu, and tae kwon do. His intense, dark eyes under heavy brows darted restlessly to take in everything around him. He laughed easily. Andrea and I both took to him immediately.

Andrea liked him especially. She joined his laughter. After just a few moments they were laughing together like old friends, and she was giving him her best, deepest, sexiest laugh as they compared notes about growing up in Queens. He was from St. Albans, which, though miles away in character from Forest Hills, was not that far in distance. They were the same age, and for a moment I felt shut out by their shared perceptions and instant compatibility. I felt like a visitor from another planet.

The feeling didn't last long. I reminded myself that if Andrea liked Robins, she would buy into the program. Her enthusiasm in a strong doctor-patient relationship would work to her benefit. And her judgment about people was inevitably good; if she liked Robins, he would be a strong, trustworthy ally. I didn't know until later, when Joanna told me, that Andrea found Robins devastatingly handsome.

The talk, in any case, soon turned to her condition. Andrea produced the test results Bob had sent with her. We both felt the urgency to get her into the program. I forced myself to hold back while she talked, not wanting to make this into a doctor's meeting, and to keep her in the loop and in control.

Soon, Robins took her to be examined. She had to repeat the stress test and some of the blood tests. We waited in a small office lounge afterward for what seemed an interminable time.

Andrea sat in quiet agitation. She closed her eyes and tried to meditate, but at last her anxiety overflowed. "I think I'll get in, Sid. I think I will, don't you?" she said. "The tests are going to be fine and he'll let me in. I just have a feeling."

"You'll get in," I assured her.

She was so afraid of being disappointed. Hyperthermia was a long shot, but in its very inconclusiveness lay the hope for cure. Schmidt had primed her to believe in the possibility, and now I was afraid she thought Dr. Robins could work wonders. He *had* been optimistic and upbeat. But he knew, as I did, that the statistics for her cancer weren't encouraging. They said it was incurable and that the probability of a long remission, let alone a cure, was remote. Robins had tried to inject reality when he told her, "Even if I can accept you, I don't promise miracles."

The doctor reappeared at last. Andrea took my hand. Robins was smiling.

"Good news," he said. "The stress test turned out fine. I've also looked over the prior results, and I'm satisfied. Congratulations."

Andrea was in. We looked at each other with a mixture of elation and relief, as if we had aced a tough exam, or been accepted into Harvard, instead of a rigorous cancer treatment trial in which all the patients, according to the trial's requirements, had advanced or metastatic cancer "with no probability of cure."

"It didn't hurt that Sid made it clear that his role is entirely as the spouse," Robins added.

I was glad I had kept my mouth shut, but there was no time to celebrate. "When can I start?" Andrea said.

"I'll admit you this afternoon. You'll have the first treatment tomorrow morning."

We filled out the usual reams of paperwork, and Andrea was shown to her room. She unpacked a few things, but there was no reason she had to stay in the hospital, so we walked around the University of Wisconsin neighborhood and campus. That evening, we ate at a restaurant near the hospital.

We both were a little nervous about her treatment, wondering silently how she would endure it. Finding it hard to talk, we devoted ourselves to studying the menu. Andrea ordered a pasta dish. She didn't usually like pasta, and I commented on it.

"If hyperthermia's supposed to be like running a marathon, I should be loading up on carbohydrates, shouldn't I?" she said. She smiled at my inability to see the obvious.

"You're right." She was making every effort to be ready when tomorrow came. I should have been getting used to her focus by now, but she continued to surprise me.

It was a short ride back to the hospital in the cold night. We sat in her room for a while, talking. Then she took out one of her books and said she needed to meditate if she was going to sleep. This time, she wanted to meditate alone. I kissed her goodnight and walked back to the inn.

Walking alone in the cold night, I realized that I already missed her. When she was in the hospital in New York, I had the children and my colleagues and my familiar surroundings to fall back on. Now, I was adrift without those anchors of familiarity. More than anything else, I knew I would miss Andrea beside me in the warmth and comfort of a shared bed. Without her, I was without a vital part. I went to sleep with a prayer in my mind and heart that hyperthermia, with all its hazards, would give her back to me.

Chapter

9

WIRES trailed from Andrea's body when I arrived at the hospital the next morning. Robins had explained that whole-body hyperthermia requires the monitoring of almost every body function. His team would track second-by-second her blood pressure, heart function, breathing, and oxygen saturation, but especially her temperature. One of an array of thermometers was at the end of a thin tube running through her nose into her esophagus, where it would allow the team to follow her internal temperature.

A nurse swabbed her arm and inserted an IV needle, then injected a sedative into the IV line.

Dr. Robins's hyperthermia unit, patented by a Menomonee Falls, Wisconsin, company and referred to as "the radiant cocoon," looked like an old-fashioned steam box. Only Andrea's head showed once she was inside and the treatment was ready to begin. She looked like the woman in the box the magician saws in half.

"Do you mind if I observe?" I asked.

"It's not a good idea," Robins said. "It's not what you expect. Frankly, it could be a little frightening."

I was surprised and somewhat concerned. I wanted to remind him I was a doctor. But he was right. I also had rejected such requests from physician-spouses of my patients. The patient requires your full attention, and the spouse can be diverting, more so if he or she gets upset. I knew it would be impossible for me to be detached where Andrea was concerned.

I retreated to her room to wait.

The treatment took three hours. I watched the clock and envisioned the phases of the treatment as Robins had described it. The nurse and a young doctor working with Robins first raised the moist, radiant heat inside the box until Andrea's body temperature reached 107.6 degrees Fahrenheit. That took sixty minutes. Then she was removed from the chamber. At that point her metabolic rate would have doubled, and, with evaporative heat losses prevented by a plastic sheet, her high temperature was maintained for another hour. The treatment was ended by removing the sheet and allowing her, over a third hour, to sweat out the heat and cool down to normal body temperature.

It was easy to imagine the stresses to which the heat subjected her. One hundred and seven point six degrees is quite high for an adult. Her face and skin would be flushed. Her heart would be racing, and every organ in her body would be working hard to cool off.

Worrier that I am, I was beginning to wonder what had gone wrong when I heard voices and a stretcher approaching down the hall. Nurses wheeled the stretcher into the room and moved the person on it, limp as a rag doll, onto the bed. I went to the bedside, but someone had made a mistake. I didn't recognize the brick red, grotesquely swollen face I saw. Its closed eyes were like pinpricks in marshmallows of flesh.

"Andrea?" I touched the flushed skin, but she didn't respond. She wasn't dead, I saw her breathing, but I thought she must be in a coma. Her legs under the sheet were twice their normal size. I looked in near-panic at the nurses.

"She's a little swollen, Dr. Winawer, but she's going to be fine," one of them said.

I remembered that she had received a lot of intravenous fluids during the treatment to keep her hydrated. Some of it escaped as sweat, more through her vascular system, but some had remained and accumulated in the tissues of her legs. The medical word for such swelling is edema.

Hours passed, and still Andrea did not respond to my touch. Her fingers, as I held her hand, were ballooned and tight as sausages. Only her slow, steady breathing told me she was still alive.

Dr. Robins appeared. "It went well," he said, detecting my worry. "She'll be fine. Fluid retention is normal with the treatment."

But he was more concerned than his confidence showed. He revealed that Andrea had been sensitive to the sedative and to other medications, too. I knew that she disliked taking drugs of any kind and would likely have had a low tolerance. Robins said he would adjust her sedative dose on the next treatment.

At last, her eyes opened. She turned to me with a great effort and her puffy features broke into a smile. She waved one of her swollen hands over her body as if waving in more medicine and said, "I got something in me. I got something in me. I got something in me." She said it over and over.

She felt something at work, some process taking place. Maybe it was the miracle we both hoped for.

I spent the rest of the day and much of the evening at her bedside. She asked for a bagel and cream cheese. I scoured the hospital and the surrounding neighborhood, and returned carrying a distant cousin of a bagel.

"We're in the land of the doughnut," I said.

She laughed and I hugged her and cried for joy that she was still with me.

We called the kids to tell them the treatment had gone well. Andrea said the worst part of it was that she couldn't get a New York bagel.

"I look like a Cabbage Patch doll," she told them. "But I know it's working. I can feel it."

T H E redness departed overnight, but not the swelling. She smiled through still-puffy features to see me the next morning.

"I'm ready to go home," she said.

"I think he wanted you to stay another day."

"What for? Let's go."

Robins reluctantly gave her an okay to travel. I walked beside my swollen angel while a skycap pushed her wheelchair through Madison's airport, and did the same thing in Milwaukee's, where we switched to a direct flight home. Andrea for a change didn't care how she looked. She was deliriously happy. She kept saying she could feel it working. She knew beyond doubt that cancer cells were being killed.

I was relieved. She had endured the treatment, first of all. And her conviction that it was working was contagious. Tests might prove otherwise, but until then, I was willing to be as convinced as she was.

Traveling at her side and feeling her confidence, I was again impressed with her. She continued to act with a rejuvenated sense of self. I was beginning to believe that her attitude alone — the force she was bringing to the direction of her treatment, and her response to it — could affect the possibility of cure. Her powerful spirit seemed actually to be capable of destroying cancer cells.

WHEN we got back to New York, Bob Kurtz asked her if she wanted to take a diuretic that would help her eliminate the excess fluid from her body. Characteristically, she said no.

"I'll get rid of it myself," she said.

Andrea believed that supplemental medications might interfere with the hyperthermia's effects. She wanted its full impact, with nothing getting in the way. She didn't want to distract her body from fighting the disease.

She was still swollen and refusing the relief of a diuretic, when Bob walked into my office. "Look at this," he said. His tone was dire and, in a way, accusing.

I scanned the paper he handed me. It contained blood test results, faxed to him by Dr. Robins. His team had drawn Andrea's blood soon after she came out of the heat chamber.

"Good lord, what's this?" I said. What I saw made me wonder, with an awful surge of guilt, if I had killed her.

The figures were scary. Her LDH was off the charts.

LDH, or lactic acid dehydrogenase, is an enzyme that exists in most if not all the cells of the body. Elevated levels of LDH usually indicate the presence of a tumor or inflammation, or other cell damage that the body is fighting. For certain types of tumors, like Andrea's, it can be an exquisitely sensitive indicator of the growth of a tumor. Andrea's LDH was running high before the hyperthermia. Consistent with her aggressive tumor, it was pushing 250, which is the upper limit of normal at Sloan-Kettering, although every patient has an individual norm.

The paper Bob had handed me showed a figure of 500.

How could I have let it happen? I wondered. The hyperthermia had been a terrible mistake.

But I couldn't be sure. LDH is also released when tumor cells are destroyed. A high LDH level can be read either way, if you're not sure what's really happening. You don't know if the glass is half empty or half full. These were the first measurable results from Andrea's treatment, and I feared the worst.

"It's utterly consistent," Dr. Robins assured us when Bob got him on the phone. "It means the hyperthermia has succeeded. Cancer cells are dying in large numbers, which is why there's a sharp and sudden rise to very high levels in the LDH. Soon it will start to fall, and we'll see levels lower than it was before the hyperthermia."

We waited.

A week after her treatment, Andrea's swelling had gone down and she looked normal. She went to the hospital to have blood drawn for a new look at her LDH.

Bob came to my office the next day, carrying a computer printout. I took it and searched for the vital LDH figure.

"Below two hundred," Bob offered.

I looked up, wanting to believe him but unsure. He smiled at my eagerness for confirmation. He said, "That's lower than before the treatment."

"That's what Robins said would happen."

"Right. It looks like it's working, Sid."

"Thank God." I turned to the printout again. I had to see it to believe it.

The results bore Robins out. The heat had stopped Andrea's rampaging cancer cells and started killing them. We didn't yet have a confirmatory CT scan, but her elevated LDH surely had been a signal of their death throes. And this was only with the heat. She hadn't yet received the chemotherapy that was a component of the treatment.

Andrea was right. Something was going on inside her body.

ANDREA needed to have an access port before she received her second treatment. Before we returned to Madison, she visited Sloan-Kettering to have one inserted.

The port is a way chemotherapy patients receive drugs without repeated puncturing of the veins that eventually can ruin them, like a needle drug addict's. It goes into the left side of the chest, high up, connecting with the subclavian vein under the collarbone. This human-made orifice is used not only for chemotherapy, but also for intravenous fluids, blood transfusions, and, if the patient needs them, other medications. It is used for taking blood for tests. Between uses, the plastic port lies under the skin forming a tiny, inconspicuous bump, ready to be accessed by a special needle through the skin and the seal at the mouth of the port.

Andrea came home with the port inserted. That night, as we got ready for bed, she stood naked in front of the mirror. Her body was softer and fuller, her ribs less starkly visible than they had been before she willed herself to eat and take in calories. The small scar from her abdominal surgery was fading. She stared at the lump formed by the port and ran her fingers over it. "I hate this," she said softly.

"I know, but it will make your treatment easier."

"I still hate it."

"You hardly see it. Nobody will know it's there."

"I can feel it. I know it's there. You know what it feels like to me, Sid?" She spun around and looked at me. "It feels like a string you tie around your finger so you don't forget something. It reminds me that I'm sick, and there's this tube going into me that shouldn't be there."

"It's just a little bump."

"It's more than just a little bump, Sid."

I stood and held her. I had seen hundreds of ports inserted and never thought about the patient's feeling of disfigurement. To me as a doctor, it was simply a convenience for the patient. With Andrea's reaction opening my eyes, I saw it now as a foreign object, an invasion of her body. She was young and kept her beauty naturally. She used body oils and a minimum of soap and makeup. The port was one more of the indignities from which women suffer in greater measure than most men, breast cancer being chief among them. I felt sad to see it and to see her reaction. "I know," I said. "I'm saying it's just a little bump to me. You're still my Number One Baby."

She relaxed in my arms. "Thanks, Sidney Jerome."

The familiar endearment told me I had found a way to say the right thing. We both knew she needed the port, but she also needed to feel it didn't detract from her or mark her as a victim.

The more time I spent on the patient side, the more I realized how much attention doctors need to pay to the associations that a patient makes. A port that made things easier for us created fallout I never had considered.

W E packed to go back to Madison. A third blood test showed Andrea's LDH had plunged to 175, and she was eager for the next stage.

This time, along with the tender mercies of the radiant heat chamber, during the twenty minutes when the temperature was highest she received an infusion of a toxic chemical dripping through the port into her bloodstream.

The chemical was carboplatin. Cisplatin, the principal agent used in the Mayo Clinic protocol, was a related platinum-based agent. However, cisplatin was too hard on the kidneys to be used in conjunction with hyperthermia, which also could cause kidney damage. Carboplatin, just as strong, did not cause kidney damage. Robins's trial had reached the stage where he was giving the drug in high doses, and the heat was multiplying its effects.

Andrea again was comatose and swollen when the nurses brought her from the treatment. As before, she woke after several hours with a smile.

It faded quickly. "Whoa," she said, grabbing her stomach as she felt one of chemotherapy's most distressing side effects. She controlled the nausea after a few moments, and smiled again, cautiously. "It's good, Sid," she said. "I can feel it. I can really feel it."

"I can see that."

"No, I mean I can feel it working."

We returned to New York the next day. Now I was anxious for a CT scan that would confirm what her LDH levels indicated. I wanted to see the cancer's shrinkage. She had the scan a day or two after we returned. In the meantime, the blood drawn after the second treatment revealed a still-dropping LDH level of 160. When Bob called to say he had the film, I was almost afraid to look at it.

I waited with trepidation while he slipped two sheets of film into the retainers at the edges of the viewing box and flipped the switch. The half-moon shape of the human liver appeared against the light on each, and, on one, the large Swiss cheese–size spots of tumor. The tumor spots were much smaller on the other.

"This is the new one, right?" I said with my voice trembling.

Bob put an arm around my shoulders and gave me a rough, indulgent squeeze. "That's right. It's still a little early, but it looks as if she may be heading toward remission."

The third stage of Robins's protocol called for chemotherapy alone. For this, we could stay in New York. Andrea checked into Memorial

Sloan-Kettering and received the chemo from her medical oncologist, Fry Casper.

Her next CT scan showed still more improvement.

THE cancer's retreat gave us permission to relax a little. The morbid cloud that had hung over our family since Andrea's diagnosis lifted just a bit. Around the apartment, the atmosphere brightened; Daniel was no less sensitive to his mother's moods, but now he joked less desperately as he saw her able to laugh easily again. Jonathan felt able to spend more time at his dormitory and less at home, and Joanna's sense of drama returned to normal levels.

Andrea announced one day when I came home that she had decided to take a job. She had not worked outside the home since before Daniel was born, when she worked as a roving teacher of deaf children in the New York City public schools. This had strained our relationship as our kids grew older and needed less attention. I wanted her to make a life for herself outside the family. She had never responded to my urging.

"Can you do that?" I said, scarcely able to believe yet another new side to her development. "With us having to go out to Wisconsin?"

"It's just three days a week," she said. "Dr. Sherman said I could work around my schedule."

Dr. Ray Sherman had an internal medicine practice on East 70th Street. He had hired Andrea to type his office notes. She took pride in her new job. It would prove to be a distraction from the cancer, a new outlet for her energy, and the focus outside the family I had hoped she could find.

Just as our laughter was returning, bad news arrived from a different quarter. Andrea's sister, Marsha, called to say their mother's fatigue, which had persisted after the Blooms had returned to Florida following Andrea's operation, had been traced to leukemia. She had received blood transfusions, and the Blooms were making plans to come to New York so that Helen could enter treatment at Sloan-Kettering.

Andrea reacted with a mixture of conflicting feelings. She had grown closer to Marsha since her diagnosis; they had never been great pals before, but now they talked on the phone almost every day. But her relationship with her mother remained turbulent. "It's the story of my life," she said, anger and disappointment in her voice. "I feel bad for her, but what about me? When I need her, where is she? Where was she ever?"

Chapter

10

I T was still only March. The days since Andrea's cancer was discovered had passed with whirlwind speed. It was only in the relative calm of her improvement that I recognized all the changes that had been taking place.

Beyond her emerging power, there was simply the intensity with which we lived. It seemed incredible that the cancer should be responsible for restoring this aspect of our lives. Yet that is how it seemed. We had been measured and predictable, with plenty of time to plan ahead systematically. Now we were scrambling for life with an accelerated timetable and a renewed spirit of adventure.

We started to explore more deeply the benefits of meditation. I had gone from an impatient observer to an enthusiastic convert as I felt my own stress evaporate under its effects. We meditated now not just to escape uncertainty and fear, but to apply our minds to healing.

This was a reverse of the previous process. The visual meditations had been conscious efforts to find a place away from the cancer. Now we were turning inward to focus on our bodies rather than distract ourselves.

We sat together, often facing each other on the bed or on the sofa in the living room. Sometimes we held hands, lightly, often just touching each other's fingertips. We closed our eyes and relaxed by concentrating on our breathing, using deep breaths to bring us to a focal point and fill ourselves with new energy.

Distracting thoughts were no longer to be avoided. We let them enter our minds, wash over us, and dissipate. We attempted to relax our muscles one by one, starting with our scalps and progressing downward through the body to the tips of our toes. We didn't follow *Gray's Anatomy,* but tried to deal with the muscles and organs as areas of the body and relax those parts. We focused thoughtfully on what was going on inside our bodies. This washed away distractions that kept wanting to take over, and allowed us to relax. I found the effect astounding; in the thinking, tension literally flowed out and disappeared.

At times I felt as if the calming signals our minds sent out encircled us both in a halo of energy. I thought of Brownian movement, in which particles suspended in a liquid or gas move not purely from their own energy, but from their interaction with other particles around them. I began to believe in the energy that some say emanates from our bodies and surrounds us. Maybe that is what we felt. We were particles moving in a force field generated by our minds. The more deeply we became integrated with our bodies, the more we felt this force.

The only distraction we couldn't avoid was Joanna, who once or twice came in to find us meditating in the living room and complained that we were getting weird. I would have thought so, too. Now I wanted more of it.

We found new and different meditations aimed at patients. One was designed to help a patient accept medicine more effectively. Andrea said she had read it in the hospital before her first session with hyperthermia and chemotherapy. In the wake of the chemo-only session in New York, she asked me to read it to her as a way of urging the toxins to keep working. It described how the medicine was given, its anatomical course through the bloodstream, through every organ of the body, and its attack and destruction of each cancer cell. She said it helped her embrace the medicine. She felt it provided greater acceptance of the treatment by her body, lessened its side effects, and increased her confidence in the outcome.

We discovered meditations aimed at connecting with other people who were healing. We read these, out loud and silently, as ways to share the burden of the cancer and to find a feeling of comfort in oneness with others. They made us — patient and spouse — feel we were not alone. We joined forces with all who were afflicted and challenged, and formed together a strong army.

In the months to come, I would begin to see these meditations as a form of prayer.

Andrea, by herself, began using a meditation technique called guided imagery. This was a way of creating an event by imagining it. She pictured the destruction of cancer cells within her body. She saw them being gobbled up by healthy white blood cells, much the way Pac-Man gobbled up its targets in the old video game. She even asked me for magnified pictures of white cells and cancer cells, so she could visualize the process realistically.

Such effects have never been proved. But meditation in all its aspects, for many, is its own reward. Andrea and I certainly found that to be true, as we realized it brought greater peace and more enjoyment to our daily lives. The major effect of meditation, and one that does seem to have provable anticancer effects, is in reducing stress.

Science has known for years that stress can cause many diseases, or certainly aggravate them. It can affect heart rate, blood pressure, and other physiological functions. But it also has a profound effect on the immune system. Stress impairs the immune system's ability by suppressing T lymphocytes, or T cells, which inactivate or destroy foreign substances. A type of T cell called the natural killer cell is especially compromised by stress, and it is these natural killer cells that attack free radicals — the molecules from fat and other substances that are suspected of a role in causing cancer.

Immunologist Ronald Glaser and his psychologist wife, Jane Kiecole-Glaser, studied the effects of stress on medical students at Ohio

State University during final exams. They learned that the stress of exams caused noticeable declines in natural killer cell activity. It also altered the ratio of two other types of T lymphocytes — helper T cells and suppressor T cells — and suppressed interferon, a family of natural proteins that suppress or destroy tumor cells and stimulate the immune system. One of the triggers lies in the pituitary gland. At the first hint of stress, the pituitary releases adrenocorticotropic hormone, or ACTH, which in turn stimulates a flood of cortisol from the adrenal glands, which sit atop each kidney. Tests have shown this hormone to depress the immune system in animals. Stress also affects the body through other physiological functions such as nerve transmission.

Stress reduction, by whatever means, can be a lifesaver. It can both prolong life and make shortened lives more meaningful.

Dr. David Spiegel at Stanford, for example, showed that women with breast cancer had a longer survival if, in addition to their standard treatment, they received psychological support that reduced stress. Memorial Sloan-Kettering's Psychiatry Department demonstrated that a version of post-traumatic stress syndrome often follows a diagnosis of cancer and a prescription of treatment, especially a very stressful treatment like bone marrow transplantation. This terrible anxiety is not so different from the post-traumatic stress seen in Vietnam War troops. This stress is so severe that it can interfere with patients' accepting and continuing with treatment. The studies show that patients accept treatment, have fewer side effects, and generally do better if their stress can be reduced.

Conversely, stress reduction through such methods as meditation can provide patients with a more receptive attitude for treatment, reduce side effects, and even reduce complications.

Studies in addition to Spiegel's suggest that reduced stress can improve survival in patients under treatment.

This evidence by now is so persuasive it cannot be denied, and it must not be ignored. Science can develop effective treatments through biological, genetic, and chemical research, but their value will be wasted if patients are not prepared to receive them. I was rethinking my textbook knowledge of the brain, seeing it less as a separate anatomic and physiological entity that acts as a control room for the body than as a far more integrated mechanism. Its role in our behavior, outlook, and capacities is an area of unmined potential. As I watched Andrea cope with her cancer by using the power of her mind, and as I experienced its effects myself in meditation, I understood that we physicians must do far more to help patients prepare themselves to receive the benefits of conventional medicine.

Encouragement and empathy are not enough. These are important, standard-issue bedside manner tools that have always been important. But I was shifting to a more activist position, seeing that we must try to give patients the psychological tools to help themselves. At some level, they must be self-empowered and independent of us, in ways that will allow them perhaps to change the course of their disease moment by moment and day by day.

ANDREA and I returned to Madison in April. By now, my sense of isolation had eased. I no longer felt so acutely the anxiety of separation from the familiar surroundings of Sloan-Kettering and the colleagues I knew and trusted. I still had them to fall back on; Robins coordinated every move in Andrea's case with physicians at Sloan-Kettering, and Bob Kurtz remained her primary doctor. But I was beginning to get used to the Midwest. I was becoming less a creature of my institution.

The fourth step in Robins's protocol repeated the second; Andrea received hyperthermia and chemotherapy in combination. Afterward, the spots on her liver were still smaller. Her LDH continued to drop as well, finding her norm of between 150 and 160. Robins was cautiously pleased.

The CT scans provided a graphic view of her improvement, but they could not be done as often as blood tests. Her LDH became the measure that we most relied on. Each blood test was accompanied by anxiety. I would check the computer every fifteen minutes until the results were posted, and then call her. I died a thousand deaths waiting for those results.

Bob Kurtz caught me one day checking the results on my computer. "Sid, you've got to cut that out," he said. "You're not her doctor. It's just not appropriate."

He was right. I was still participating too actively in her case, rather than simply trying to support her. But I couldn't stop. I had to know. And it was as if, by tapping the keys and clicking the mouse of the computer, I could will it to give a good result.

As the string of good results continued, I was thrilled. The blood tests and the pictures of the shrinking tumor blasted away my doubts about hyperthermia as a summer squall erases clouds and leaves blue sky. Andrea's progress so far probably would have happened with the Mayo Clinic cisplatin protocol. She had not received cancer-killing drugs before, and was sensitive to them. But the hyperthermia plus chemo did it with a minimum of side effects. Andrea's swelling went away reasonably soon, and she suffered little nausea from the chemo. The hyperthermia, as Robins's studies showed, must have enhanced the chemotherapy's ability to attack the cancer cells without harming natural cells. As evidence, Andrea still had her hair, one of the first casualties of traditional chemotherapy.

We had to remind ourselves to be cautious. I, especially, knew that cancer often retreated under an initial onslaught, disappeared for a time, and then came back in full fury. Hers had not yet fully disappeared. But it was tempting, despite the positive changes we had made, to imagine our old life back. Life with its ordinary daily pleasures, free of the threat that was transforming us. A life that would restore the sense that we had time to anticipate slow days growing old together.

"Don't think like that," Schmidt warned. "It's dangerous. It could even be fatal. It is backsliding down the hill again."

"What's wrong with wanting to be free of cancer?" Andrea asked. We had gone to see him together on a Saturday afternoon to share our growing optimism.

"There is nothing wrong with wanting to be free of cancer. There is very much wrong with wanting to be free of its concerns."

"What's the difference?" I said. I couldn't understand why the psychiatrist couldn't allow us to feel good about the way things were going.

"You have been doing some very positive things. Making changes that are working to your benefit. If you are not worried, it will turn you around to where you were before. For you, Andrea, that means a return to the feelings your mother gave you in your childhood. You were not worthy of attention. That's why you had to be at death's door before you could do things that were beneficial to yourself, like eat. Only by fighting for your life could you deserve these things."

"Wait a minute," I said after Schmidt's meaning filtered through to me. "Are you saying that's why Andrea got cancer?"

"That's certainly one interpretation, yes."

"That's wrong. That's just wrong. It's cruel," I protested.

Schmidt had bought fully into the theory of the cancer personality. This theory was nothing new. It had been around since Galen, the ancient Greek physician, observed that melancholy women were more likely to get breast cancer. The theory fell out of favor with the advance of surgery and radiation therapy after the turn of the century. It was revived by Lawrence LeShan, the psychologist and psychotherapist whose books on meditation we had read and admired. LeShan, with colleague Richard Worthington, had interviewed 250 cancer patients and narrowed down their common traits: almost 80 percent felt self-dislike or self-distrust; 64 percent were unable to express hostility; 38 percent felt tension from their relationship with one or both parents; and over three-fourths had lost someone close, such as a spouse or a child, before the cancer was diagnosed. LeShan wrote that most cancer patients had, among other psychological markers, childhoods or teen years marked by feelings of isolation. They were contemptuous of themselves, their abilities and personalities. Cancer patients are "empty of feeling and devoid of self," he wrote, and those who didn't respond to treatment had lost hope of having meaningful lives.

In *Illness as Metaphor*, Susan Sontag pointed to such views as "preposterous and dangerous." They not only put the onus of the disease on the patient, but the burden of cure on the patient's ability to find a self-love he or she supposedly lacked in the first place.

"I only said it's one interpretation," Schmidt said. Andrea's raised hand stopped me from saying any more. Her belief in the mind's powers aligned her more with Schmidt's and LeShan's point of view. It had allowed her to take responsibility for a role in fighting the cancer. I worried that her ability to bear that responsibility would be undercut by also shouldering the blame.

I drove home fuming. Andrea tried to calm me. "He only said we shouldn't go back. That's all. I don't think I gave myself cancer."

All the same, I thought it was unconscionable for any doctor to place the blame for the disease on the victim. People smoke and eat themselves to death, and other people who do nothing unhealthy are struck by disease. Diet, lifestyle, environment, heredity, and random mutations all enter into the mix of the things that happen to all of us, every day. Psychologists and psychiatrists who attribute cancer solely to personality, or to stress and its handling by certain personality types, overlook these factors. Once again, I felt the profound ambivalence that had marked my relationship with Schmidt. There was no denying that he had helped us identify our problems. But since Andrea's cancer he had seemed preternaturally interested in both her course of treatment and the psychological touchstones of her cancer. It was almost as if she mirrored something in himself, that he saw his destiny as tied to hers. Why this might be I didn't know, but it made me think that, sometimes, his influence on her was far too strong.

His next suggestion for her treatment threw a monkey wrench into Andrea's hyperthermia regimen and threw me into an ethical dilemma.

Chapter

11

INTERFERON? You want her to take interferon?"

I gawked at Schmidt. A week had passed since he had seemed to blame Andrea for the personality that caused her cancer. She had three sessions left in the hyperthermia protocol, and spring was breaking out all over in New York. I sat up on the edge of my chair.

He nodded in his deliberate way. "I've talked about it with someone. I think it could help."

"Could help? What's going on?" I protested. "She's in a program that you introduced us to. It seems to be working. She's doing well, with minimal side effects. Why should she change anything?"

I had barely gotten used to Andrea's receiving hyperthermia, with the positive test results melting my initial fears; now Schmidt wanted to add a new ingredient. To alter a medical trial protocol in such a way is outside the bounds of accepted medical practice. Just as I was getting my footing, the ground was shifting again under my feet.

"Dr. Winawer, I know the hyperthermia is working," he said. The professional formality with which he had first addressed me nine years earlier had never changed. "But Andrea is in a terrible war. She is fighting for her life. Her cancer is aggressive and lethal, as you know. The hyperthermia and chemotherapy may cause a remission, but the cancer may come back. Small doses of interferon, taken once a month, will help her immune system to fight it. It would be a mopping-up operation, a way of getting the cancer cells the big guns miss."

Not only had Schmidt embraced psychotherapy's view of the cancer personality, he had embraced the metaphors that had grown up around cancer. I was guilty, too. It was easy to think and speak of cancer as "the enemy," of its presence in the body as an "invasion" or an "assault," and of its treatments as "counterattacks." Susan Sontag argued that such terms discourage patients and often dissuade them from seeking treatment. It was the rare patient who was fully prepared to "fight back" when theories of the cancer personality told patients their lack of self-worth had caused the problem in the first place. Andrea, however, seemed to be doing it.

"But what you're suggesting is totally unproven. It's never been done, as far as I know," I protested. I knew Ian Robins had used interferon with hyperthermia, but at much higher doses combined with a lower body temperature, and without chemotherapy. "Have you discussed this with her?"

Schmidt, sitting with one leg draped across the other, nodded. Outside the window behind him, the trees of Riverside Park were beginning to bud. Traffic sounds came up faintly from the street four floors below.

In a sudden fury at Schmidt's manipulation of my wife, and his drawing me into something I wanted no part of, I lashed out at him. "Are you nuts? Just what the hell are you trying to pull?"

The psychiatrist displayed no emotion at my outburst. "It's only a suggestion," he said calmly.

"Who will administer it? Who will prescribe it? What doctor? I'm certainly not going to."

"Well, I know somebody."

"Who, who do you know who would do this, knowing she's part of a trial protocol? Do we tell Dr. Robins? Do we tell Dr. Kurtz? Or are we supposed to hide this from them? How do you handle the effects?"

"I know a doctor in Atlanta. He's a reputable man, and he has experience with this kind of treatment." He ignored the other questions.

"We're flying to Wisconsin once a month for hyperthermia. Now you want us to fly to Atlanta for interferon shots?"

"It's only a suggestion," he repeated. "It's entirely up to you and Andrea." His tone softened. "Try to have an open mind. Read up on it. Call the doctor, here's his number. You'll find a great deal of evidence in its favor. You may find enough to persuade you it's not a bad idea."

At that moment I felt like I wanted to kill him. I felt trapped, as if he had a thumb to my head and was pressing me between the jaws of a vice. On one hand was my conventional medical perspective, on the other, my growing understanding of the patient's need to believe in something more. What's more, it was a situation I couldn't get out of. Having accepted Andrea's wish for hyperthermia, I could not very well turn rigid now. I hated Schmidt's arrogance. But I knew I would help Andrea if a shred of evidence supported his suggestion and that was what she wanted.

There was no question by now whose decision it would be.

HATING myself for being so pliable, but telling myself I was helping Andrea, I began a search.

I was developing a routine for the searches. First I picked a search term to cover all the bases. In this case it was "Interferon in Cancer Treatment." I submitted it to the medical librarian with a request for all human and animal studies in the last five years. The librarian's computerized inquiry to Medline, a medical database, produced stacks of abstracts and summaries of research papers. From these I decided which full papers I wanted to review. When the subject was hyperthermia, I discussed significant findings with Andrea and the doctors on her case, including Dr. Schmidt. I didn't plan to discuss interferon with anyone but Andrea and Dr. Schmidt.

After a day or two, I reluctantly admitted to myself that Schmidt wasn't that far off in his thinking.

The protein molecules of the interferon family are manufactured by white blood cells (lymphocytes) in response to viral infections or to various substances that will stimulate them. Interferons act by binding to a receptor on the surface of a cell. This produces a series of events within the cell: viruses are inhibited from reproducing, cell reproduction is suppressed, the immune system within the cell is stimulated to secrete cytokines, and lymphocytes attack cancer cells, viruses, and bacteria with greater vigor.

At the time of my search, the biology of all this was still unfolding. Interferon apparently attacked certain tumors and destroyed cancer cells by simultaneously exciting the body's immune activity and slowing down cell reproduction. This had led to its use, in conjunction with other drugs, against several types of cancers, especially Kaposi's sarcoma, which is associated with AIDS. And it was being used by itself to treat viral hepatitis.

I was more encouraged when studies came across my desk showing that interferon had been used successfully against carcinoid tumors like Andrea's. They were slow-growing, however, not the aggressive type she had. In those cases, the interferon was administered by injection in large doses, at least three to five times weekly.

One study was by a group in Uppsala, Sweden, a beautiful old university town Andrea and I once visited while I attended a medical conference. Dr. Kjell Oberg's team had more experience with this than any of the others I found. His group had treated patients with doses of three to six million units of interferon daily for up to two years. Almost half the patients experienced tumor shrinkage. Others stabilized for two years without tumor growth. It wasn't a cure, but it was a good result with any single drug.

I was excited to see that two of the patients had experienced a complete remission, with all signs of the tumor gone.

One of the oncologists at Sloan-Kettering also informed me about a protocol in which interferon was used along with other chemotherapeutic drugs to treat neuroendocrine cancers like Andrea's. This was a last-ditch effort, though, and the interferon, again, was used in large doses.

Schmidt's suggestion of a series of three doses once a month was a fraction of any dosage that had been effective as a primary treatment.

With all this information in hand, and new questions every minute, I decided to talk with Dr. Lloyd Old, a brilliant, world-respected immunologist who was working at Sloan-Kettering. Dr. Old put me in touch with Dr. Oberg in Sweden. I reviewed with him Andrea's case and her treatment. "Someone suggested we look into interferon. What do you think?"

"Well, we don't have any experience with such small doses. I don't think it would do her any good, but I can't say that for sure. I don't think it would do her any harm."

But I also learned from the papers that came across my desk and the doctors I spoke with that a number of potentially dangerous side effects had been observed with interferon. The least of these was a flu-like syndrome that left patients weak and achy. It could create problems with liver function, reduce the blood cell population by depressing the bone marrow, or overstimulate the immune system, causing the body to produce antibodies against its own tissues, especially the thyroid gland, with resulting inflammation. Studies reported a lupus-like reaction as a result of all the antibodies being stimulated by the interferon. This outpouring of antibodies could cause an autoimmune syndrome, in which normal cells were attacked and destroyed.

I LAID these findings out to Andrea in our living room/war room, with Daisy on the couch beside her. "It's a two-edged sword," I said. "The idea has potential, but the downside could be horrible."

The medical papers on the large, low coffee table had multiplied. The papers on hyperthermia were buried under the results of new searches. We had been doing this almost every night after dinner, pouring over possible new ways to treat her cancer. Books on meditation were a part of the pile, as we continued exploring different meditations. Shirley would stack everything neatly, and we would mess it up again. Tonight a Brahms symphony was playing in the background.

"Besides, you can't just add drugs to a protocol without knowing what they'll do," I added.

"Dr. Schmidt says it could help."

"Why do you want to do everything he says?" I grumbled.

"He just wants to help. Come on, Sid, he's helped us a lot. You know that."

She had put her finger on my ambivalence about Schmidt. He had helped us work out the differences within our family. That was why I could never dismiss him out of hand. But this was medical advice of a far different sort. I returned to ground where I was comfortable.

"It could help, I suppose," I said. "But there's no proof of that. Especially only three times a month."

"There's no proof it doesn't," she replied stubbornly.

"It could interfere with your progress from the hyperthermia and chemo."

"It might not."

"Maybe your blood counts will go down."

"Maybe they won't."

"There could be a rebound effect. The cancer could come back stronger than ever."

"That could happen anyway."

"There are side effects."

"I've lived through side effects."

"What is Robins going to think? It would violate his protocol. Adding a drug like interferon is a violation of every medical principle I know. This is full-blown alternative medicine we're getting into, if somebody's going to prescribe it knowing a patient's in a protocol. Robins would kick us out of the hyperthermia program, and he'd be right to do it."

"He'd kick me out, not you." Andrea rose and walked to the other side of the coffee table, where she turned to face me. "Sid, I understand your feelings. You're a good doctor and a good man, and I love you and I know you love me and want to help me. I understand your medical concerns. I understand the relationship you have with your colleagues. You had a hard time with hyperthermia at first, remember? Sidney Jerome. I know this is a problem for you. But I have this terrible tumor.

It may kill me. I have to do everything I can. So I'm going to get it anyway. I'll go to see this doctor in Atlanta by myself."

W E made plans to go to Atlanta.

I would never in a thousand years have dreamed of violating the protocols of Robins's trial if Andrea had not insisted, and if I had not loved her as I did. Trial protocols are inviolable; only with the careful data records they provide can conclusions about their effectiveness be made and guidelines for treatment drawn.

That was the thought of the doctor and researcher. On the patient side, I rationalized that trials are always slow. The dying have no time for research. Of course, they benefit from research. Without it, medicine would have no proven weapons. But when a life is at stake, the life of someone you love, you want to pull out all the stops. Throw every weapon you can get your hands on at a disease, and in the end, if the patient lives, who cares what worked and what didn't. Emotion rules, sweeping aside valid considerations about what painstaking research may tell us about benefit and risk.

That was how much I had changed, how much my transformation had progressed. Andrea was the patient. I was the spouse. Of the two claims on me, the one I really cared about was hers. I was putting one foot in front of the other. I would take the next step, whatever it was, when we got there.

Chapter

12

DANIEL drove Andrea to LaGuardia Airport for an early morning flight to Atlanta. She wanted to spend some time with her friend Judy Fineberg, and get away from me and my agitation about the prospect of her taking interferon. I was trying to keep an open mind, but it was hard. I still didn't know what I would do when it got down to the event. I was going to see the patients I had scheduled, wrap up some paperwork, and fly down the next day.

They picked me up at the airport and we went to Judy's house and then to Stone Mountain Park, a granite mountain where the busts of Confederate leaders are carved in a Southern version of Mount Rushmore. Spring was in full bloom, and Andrea kept exclaiming about the riot of pink and white dogwoods and azaleas. She enjoyed the park's gift shop, with its little jars of condiments all tied up in bows. I tried to join her enthusiasm, but I couldn't get my mind off the real purpose of our trip. It was a relief when we finally left for her appointment.

She and Judy talked and laughed on the way. They had been roommates at Boston University. Judy, a radiologist, was the premed student Andrea often had joined for meals at the cafeteria at Boston City Hospital when I was there. They had stayed in close touch over the years. Now, they might have been attending a reunion, enjoying each other's company without a care in the world, while I brooded in the back seat about Andrea's new experiment in cancer treatment.

The doctor Schmidt had recommended worked out of a modest office complex near the airport. I was surprised when we arrived to learn that he was a clinical pathologist and that the building was mainly a reference laboratory. A receptionist called him and pointed the way to a clinical area tucked away in the back.

The doctor greeted us with a smile and invited us into his small office. Short and thin, he reminded me of a rose bush that had been trimmed too much. His thick mustache, salt-and-pepper like his wavy hair, seemed to overwhelm his features.

Although he was a clinical pathologist, he clearly had experience with patients. His manner was calm and professional. He explained that he had been doing clinical work a long time, as part of an ad hoc group that had pushed for new AIDS treatments. He said he had experimented with whole-body hyperthermia, primarily in Europe. I found myself liking him against all the odds of his recommendation by Schmidt and my reluctance to stray from the norms of cancer treatment. Andrea seemed to like him, too, and as usual I counted her judgment as a mark in his favor. He looked over her pathology report, asked a few questions about her medical history, and then took her into an examining room.

Judy and I talked while we waited. In the strange surroundings, again on the verge of a medical decision that went against the grain, I suppose I started feeling burdened, and idle chat gave way to a torrent of emotion. I told her how much I loved Andrea, and the shock the cancer and its devastating prognosis had dealt to us, the children, and our plans. I cried, while Judy listened sympathetically. My anguish was raw and my desolation real. Those feelings were as central to being a patient's spouse as my determination to support her. But if they overwhelmed me, they could defeat us both. Our partnership stood on working together, in the same direction. To relocate my own empowerment and bring it into phase with hers, I forced myself to think about Andrea's improvement and her progress toward remission.

I had composed myself when the doctor brought Andrea back from the examining room. "I've been talking with Casper Schmidt about your case," he said. "He's told me about the background of eating disorder. I'm going to suggest some antioxidant-rich vitamin supplements, a regular program of nutrition, and aspirin."

He started making out a list. The aspirin, he said, would block enzyme systems necessary for cells to stick together. The idea was that by altering cellular adhesion it might block metastatic tumors. Suddenly I had the insight that Schmidt's cancer treatment theories came from an AIDS sensibility. Desperate to combat that awful scourge, patients and sympathetic doctors pushed to see promising theories put into practice before research proved them out. I wondered about Schmidt's connection to AIDS and to this doctor who seemed to be pushing the limits of its treatment. I suspected he had AIDS patients in his practice, and in counseling them had encountered the treatments he was suggesting that Andrea consider.

I realized I felt no different when it came to treating her: promise equaled hope. The proof could wait.

"Now," he said, "we know that in your case there are no permanently effective drugs. So what can we do immunologically to sustain a response? You're receiving hyperthermia. I think interferon is appropriate to further stimulate the immune system. It will enhance the antigen presentation, remove the tumor's mask, so to speak, and allow the body to more efficiently recognize the abnormality in the tumor versus normal cells. Giving it in a pulse method, three closely spaced shots once a month, will perturb the immune system to an enhanced level of cytotoxic cell killing."

Seeing the amusement on my face and Andrea's blank expression, he laughed and continued using slightly less doctor-speak. "The idea is to get the body to recognize its tumor and produce a specific immune reaction that will maintain the tumor in check."

He scribbled a prescription and handed it across the desk. "Here's a prescription. I'll administer the first shot. Dr. Winawer, I assume you'll do it after that." He smiled, probably realizing that like most doctors I hadn't given a shot in years. "I'll show you how."

"Wait," I said. "You're sure there's nothing that will interfere with the hyperthermia?"

"Nothing. If anything, it will enhance it."

"Will it be detectable in blood tests?"

"She'll receive it midway between sessions in order to work separately, at a time when the chemotherapy's effects on her bone marrow subside, so I shouldn't think so."

"What about side effects?" I asked.

He downplayed them, saying that Andrea would have a fever but it would subside and there would be no other significant side effects.

Andrea and I followed him to the examining room. I was resigned now. We were going ahead. The doctor prepared a syringe and injected six million units of interferon into the muscle on one side of her buttocks. I knew from my research that, by contrast, interferon given for Kaposi's sarcoma was administered in fifty-million-unit doses. He followed the interferon with an injection, into her upper arm, of a naturally occurring human hormone called somatostatin.

I actually had high hopes for the somatostatin, which Schmidt also had suggested. My flurry of research had turned up studies in France and England as well as the United States that showed it sometimes slowed or halted the growth of carcinoid tumors. It also normally maintained the body's equilibrium by acting as a brake on other hormones. I found studies in which somatostatin analogues were being tested, as well as somatostatin in conjunction with chemicals or cytotoxic antibodies that could destroy cancer cells once the somatostatin hooked onto receptors in a tumor. Andrea's tumor was rich in somatostatin receptors, according to an analysis by Dr. Jean Claude Rubei at the Sandoz Research Institute in Bern, Switzerland. He was one of the few people in the world who could analyze for the presence of these receptors. After Andrea had surgery, I had sent him specimens of the tumor, frozen on dry ice, in the hope that he would find them, although aggressive neuroendocrine carcinomas generally have few if any.

None of the studies I turned up were ready for testing against Andrea's tumor. None so far had even turned out to be effective. Nonetheless, I felt injections of somatostatin with the interferon would increase the body's natural dose. It gave us one more weapon.

J U D Y drove us to a motel near the airport. It was a middle-of-the-road motel, the kind where business people stay, but it made everything seem more sleazy and desperate, like some kind of secret assignation. It went with giving Andrea the interferon and not telling Robins. Judy stayed until Andrea put on her big black T-shirt, signaling that she was going into treatment mode. Then she gave us each a hug and wished us good luck.

Andrea crawled into one of the two double beds, ready for the fever.

Night fell, and Andrea's temperature started to climb. Her face flushed. Soon she started to sweat. As the fever rose steadily higher, she tossed on the bed and pushed away the covers. I put cold towels on her face and neck, but they failed to cool her, and she shook them off and pushed me away. Watching her, I grew frightened. I felt sure she was going to have a seizure and die.

A doctor can come up with more potential problems than any layman can ever imagine. I knew in my heart and intellectually that adults don't get seizures when they run high fevers, but I was not running on intellect.

During those hours, as she writhed and her perspiration soaked the bedclothes, I didn't think of Andrea's empowerment. I didn't salute her assertiveness in taking the reins of her own treatment. I was just afraid, and not only for her but for myself also. My desire to help her had gone too far. We had crossed the line. We were both feet into alternative medicine, where disdain for established medical practice was rife. I would never be able to face my colleagues. It wasn't the interferon, but how we were using it — as an unauthorized adjunct to an approved protocol treatment, given in a manner and on a schedule that was untested. In that sense the interferon was in the worst vein of alternative medicine. We were using it behind her doctors' backs.

Andrea had become a medical outlaw. I was her sidekick, her partner in crime. We hadn't broken any laws. We had just broken the sacred rules of my profession.

She twisted and kicked away the covers. Her heat and harsh breathing seemed to fill the room. I paced the floor and wondered how I had allowed myself to get into a position where my wife was tossing with fever in a motel room without a bona fide doctor to take care of her, or even a nurse. I was not an expert in this kind of treatment and, anyway, I had no business treating her at all. Every fiber of my being screamed accusations at me for violating what I had always believed. I had gone along with her out of love, because she wanted it. But my love had been misguided. I was not medically prepared to handle complications or emergencies.

I did the only thing I could do. I waited, and prayed, and hoped for the best.

Andrea, by contrast, seemed happier with each upward tick of her temperature and each increase in discomfort. As with the hyperthermia, she felt something happening inside her to the cancer. I took her temperature every half hour. It reached 104.

There it stopped. It held there for several hours, then gradually subsided. Andrea slept. I didn't know which of us was more exhausted.

I WAS sitting in a chair by the window the next morning when Andrea opened her eyes. She looked around at the unfamiliar room and then at me. Our eyes met. She smiled as she had when she woke up after the hyperthermia.

"How are you?" she said.

"How are you? That's more important."

"I'm wet." She held her damp T-shirt away from her body. "Something happened. I'm not sure what, but something did. I feel good." She pulled the T-shirt off over her head and shook out her hair. "I feel really good. Come to bed with me."

After we showered and dressed, we walked outside into the fresh spring air. It felt scrubbed and clean after the confinement of the room. Andrea ran to the edge of the motel's parking lot to a dogwood tree in full flower. She shook a low branch, and threw back her head and laughed as its white flowers cascaded over her.

We ate breakfast at a twenty-four-hour greasy spoon next to the motel. Judy showed up soon after that to drive us to the airport.

"How did it go?" Judy asked.

"Great," said Andrea.

"I was scared," I said. Our voices overlapped. We looked at each other and laughed at the different reactions, but there was no way to describe the depth of my relief. It had been one of the most harrowing nights of my life.

Andrea slept on the plane. That night at home, using supplies of the drugs the doctor had given us to use before I filled his prescription, I prepared two syringes. Andrea lay on the bed, and I gave her eight million units of interferon with an injection in the buttocks. I winced as her flesh tensed. It hurt me to prick her with the needle. The second injection, of somatostatin, went into the upper arm and was a little easier. I closed the bedroom door, and we waited.

Her temperature rose to a fever level within hours. She smiled as it came on, and we read together one of the meditations for taking medicine. Despite the higher dose, her fever was milder than it had been the night before. Her discomfort was less, and so was mine.

I gave her ten million units the next night, according to the pulse method prescription. Again, despite the even higher dose, the fever was no worse.

T W O weeks later, April had turned to May. Andrea had celebrated her forty-sixth birthday and returned to Madison for the next session in her hyperthermia treatment. Judy Fineberg volunteered to join her, and Andrea was happy to accept though I was reluctant to let her go without me.

She was full of energy when she returned, talking about their shopping trips together. I sensed she was glad to be free of my concern for a few days.

I asked her if she had told Dr. Robins she had taken interferon.

"No," she said. "I didn't think it was important."

I held my breath waiting for the results of the next blood test. I was afraid we would be found out. But the doctor in Atlanta had been right. Either the interferon and somatostatin could not be detected in Andrea's blood, or the testing done primarily for LDH and liver function did not look for it. Our secret was safe, and we kept it to ourselves.

Her LDH continued to improve, dipping below 150. Her May CT scan also showed continued improvement. As far as we could tell, the unauthorized drugs had done no harm.

Were they a part of the good news? I didn't know. By some lights we were still on the track that could have been predicted under the Mayo Clinic protocol. Only time would tell if even the hyperthermia had made a difference. The bald truth was, I didn't care. As Andrea continued to move toward remission, each improvement lifted her spirits and mine, too. I was happy to believe the interferon was contributing.

I have to say that it was expensive. The $400 a month was covered by insurance. Here again, we were quite fortunate. Andrea wanted it, it seemed to help her, and so I resolved my doubts in favor of it. Hyperthermia, chemotherapy, interferon, somatostatin, meditation, a more nutritious diet, even her new job and increased physical activity, all of these things played a part in a new, more healthy outlook. She had devised a highly integrated program of conventional — if one could call hyperthermia conventional — and alternative treatments. Andrea's drive and my medical access and skills brought it all together. Some of it would be hard to duplicate. If a patient came to me wanting to add interferon to a conventional protocol, I would think long and hard. Interferon is strong medicine, with side effects. I don't know, even now, if it helped or hurt her. We didn't reveal its use to Robins because Andrea was afraid of his veto and thought she could handle it, but it would be safer for a patient considering interferon in conjunction with conventional cancer therapy to discuss it with his or her oncologist.

As far as Andrea was concerned, I repeated the three-injection series of interferon and somatostatin two weeks after she had returned from Madison.

Chapter

13

J U N E ' S arrival brought, along with sustained good weather that allowed us to start spending weekends at the Amagansett beach house, joy in knowing that my first dire expectation had been wrong. Five months from the onset of Andrea's pain and my initial fear that she had a typical gastric cancer, she still was a long way from dying. Despite Schmidt's admonitions, we all relaxed a little. Life in our family returned almost to normal.

With Andrea working three days a week, I picked up some of my clinical duties again. The hospital routine felt good. It was a relief seeing patients whose problems weren't my own. Growing out of my experience with Andrea, however, I found myself more attuned to them. I focused better and listened harder. I looked for signs of underlying strength or distress, and tried to play up one and alleviate the other. I often suggested to anxious patients that they try meditation and recommended Bernie Siegel's books. I paid special attention to the spouses, trying to bring them into treatment plans as much as the patients.

It was an exhilarating feeling. I felt as if I had removed a barrier between the patients and what they really needed. They, in turn, seemed grateful to be given the opportunity to discuss all aspects of their cases. They opened up with fears and feelings that in turn gave me fuller, more three-dimensional views of their cases and how to treat them.

Daniel was still at home. He was taking a light load of courses at NYU, and working part-time for one of my colleagues in the Gastroenterology Service. Jonathan was involved in campus life and final exams at Columbia, but unknown to us, he was planning to interrupt his education.

Joanna, like all teenagers her age, preferred time with her friends to time at home. She was doing well in the demanding climate of Bronx Science as she neared the end of her junior year. She was, however, troubled in a way I didn't realize until one day she approached me with a question:

"Dad, Mommy has cancer, right. And her mother has leukemia. Could I be next?"

I had to think about it. When I did, I reassured her that the statistics were very much in her favor. Although there are more than two hundred hereditary cancer syndromes that can cast an ominous shadow over a family, only 10 percent of cancers are attributed to inheritance. Andrea's family exhibited no cancer pattern. Her mother had several siblings, none of whom had cancer, and Andrea's sister, Marsha, and her children were cancer-free as well. There was no cancer pattern of known hereditary origin.

"I doubt it," I told Joanna. "Neither your grandmother's leukemia nor your mother's carcinoid tumor is inherited. They're random events, not related to each other."

W H I L E we had resumed something resembling a normal routine, each day brought evidence of the changes Andrea's cancer had brought to our household and to Andrea specifically. Her low-fat diet rich in fruits and vegetables, high in carbohydrates and low in animal protein, had become the family norm. This way, she was satisfied that she was helping prevent her cancer from returning while the rest of us were reducing our risk of cancer in the first place. We tried to keep fat to under 30 percent of the total calories in the meals we ate at home; 20 percent would have been ideal, but we weren't martyrs.

Andrea went well beyond the vitamin intake provided by her diet. She sat at the kitchen table each morning with a rainbow array of vitamin pills laid out in front of her. Schmidt, as well as the doctor in Atlanta and many alternative medicine theorists, preached that the body can be fine-tuned and balanced not only to reduce the risk of cancer but to fight cancers that already exist. The prescription we had brought home from Atlanta included beta carotene, vitamins C and E, and a special multivitamin called CO-Q10. The key, in each case, was antioxidants.

These substances and foods containing them, such as yellow, orange, and green vegetables, vitamin C–rich citrus fruits, tomatoes, and strawberries, and grain products rich in selenium, counteract the effect of molecules called free radicals.

Oxygen-free radicals are common but highly reactive substances that form as byproducts of the normal metabolism. They also can result from exposure to the sun, x-rays, tobacco, smoke, or other toxins. Free radicals can attack cell membranes and damage the cells' DNA, and lead to cancer.

Studies now estimate that a fruit and vegetable–rich diet can prevent one-third of the cancer deaths in the United States today. Foods such as tomatoes, cauliflower, broccoli, and orange juice, for example, contain hundreds of naturally occurring chemicals that are thought to provide some protection from cancer. The benefits of supplements are so far unproven.

For years the conventional view was that a healthy diet precluded the need for vitamin supplements. However, some vitamins, such as vitamin E, are hard to get sufficiently in food. Many people can't always eat a healthy, vitamin-rich diet every day, and it is hard to argue that they should do without supplements. Moreover, the RDA — recommended daily allowance — of vitamins set by the Food and Nutrition

Board of the National Academy of Sciences is based on preventing vitamin deficiencies, not on fighting cancer and other illnesses. Proponents of supplements make this point in arguing for their use, often in megadoses, but little is known about the benefits of megadose vitamins or the risks from overdose toxicity.

It does seem clear that people should eat the healthiest diet possible. Those who choose supplements should take them in addition to, not instead of, vitamins in food. Andrea, for example, took them as insurance that she was getting enough of their cancer-fighting benefits. I believe that until the role of supplements is clearer, both in preventing cancer and in helping patients recover from existing cancers, people simply should follow their convictions.

Calcium and iron pills also were part of Andrea's breakfast array. She believed the calcium would both protect against regrowth of cancer cells and strengthen her bones so she could exercise intensely without worrying about breaks and fractures. The iron counteracted her tendency to be anemic; though she ate more healthy foods than before her diagnosis, she still ate lightly.

Nevertheless, her approach to diet was a sea change, and I was delighted with it. The longstanding anorexia that had so disturbed me was less in evidence. Food was a subject that in our home had been a focus of conflict and distress. Now we were more relaxed, sound, and reasonable about it. Andrea no longer discouraged Joanna from taking second helpings. Instead, she discussed the nutritional properties of foods and rhapsodized about new taste discoveries.

Andrea's diet gave her more energy, allowing her to exercise. For years, she had not gotten much exercise at all, but as it had galvanized her in so many other ways, the cancer forced her to look at her habits and improve them.

Exercise for Andrea primarily took the form of walking. I would arrive home from the hospital to find her wearing a sweatsuit or shorts depending on the weather, waiting for me to change and join her. At first we walked leisurely, rediscovering Yorktown's shops and restaurants and street vendors, and stopping to window-shop as we held hands. Gradually, however, Andrea preferred a faster pace. She took up power walking, walking fast with her arms pumping so that we couldn't walk side by side; I had to follow her, and work hard to keep up.

I kept my schedule light and made a point of seeing that we embraced live music with the same fervor we had enjoyed after we first met. We attended operas, ballets, and symphony concerts, and I took greater joy in them than ever. The music touched deeper chords within me. It seemed more precious and more necessary.

Andrea took pleasure in the music, too. But I think that she enjoyed her new job most of all. I would come home to find her bubbling with stories of what had happened that day at Dr. Sherman's office, of her lunches and conversations with the other staff. It was clear that the job helped her keep her mind off her cancer. More important, the acceptance she found and the new life she added to the workplace built up her belief in herself and her ability to fight the cancer.

She didn't need the money that she made. She put her paychecks in a drawer and hoarded them. Then, when they totaled enough, she would announce that she was taking the family out for a good meal, or she'd surprise the kids or me with presents.

THE pile of meditation books in the living room continued to grow. Andrea was gravitating more to Larry LeShan's pioneering works on meditation and mind-body healing. While I saw in LeShan's emphasis on personality a tendency to blame the patient, she saw the opportunity to harness her mind's power to make herself well. And she liked LeShan's message that surviving is not all there is to victory, that death is not losing, or a failure, but that the winning lies in self-empowerment.

LeShan was in his seventies, but still quite active, and we took two weekends to travel to seminars he was giving in Cambridge, Massachusetts, and Princeton, New Jersey. He proved to be a big, burly, fatherly figure. At the seminars, he told stories about patients who had embraced new, zestful lives after developing cancer. Some survived and some didn't in LeShan's recounting, but all of them changed. They did things they always had wanted to do, breaking through walls of habit and improving the quality of their lives.

This part of LeShan's message hit home with me as well as Andrea. I had seen Andrea's startling emergence over the past months. Now I was beginning to see how, despite the shadow of the cancer, the changes it had caused in our lives were all for the better.

Andrea followed the seminars with an appointment with LeShan in his Manhattan office. She came home and said, "I have to reexamine my priorities. I found out I waste too much time worrying about things that don't matter very much."

"What do you mean?" I asked.

"Like at night, when people call us trying to sell something, I'm always nice to them. I want them to like me, and it takes time. I'm not going to do that anymore. And I worry about whether to buy irises or lilies to put on the piano. Who cares? They both look nice. I'm just not going to agonize anymore about those kinds of things."

She would, she said, spend her time on herself, the family, and a few good friends. She would not suffer fools or endure annoyance. She made plans to do the things that she enjoyed and swept everything else to the side.

Our meditations, influenced by LeShan, grew longer. From five or ten minutes, they stretched to thirty and forty. We continued to concentrate on breathing and relaxation of joints, muscles, and organs. As we grew more adept at eliminating mind clutter, our first forays into meditation now seemed primitive. We had been tiptoeing on a lake that had just frozen over. Now we were walking solidly in the world of meditation. Meditating together, I felt a literal physical connection of energy flowing between us. The effect was of deep sleep. Even ten or fifteen minutes of deeply concentrated meditation produced a restfulness that felt like a full night of peaceful sleeping. We opened our eyes afterward refreshed and energized.

At other times we simply read meditations to each other from selections by Bernie Siegel and Stephen Levine, another expert in the field.

Andrea continued to want me to read to her, and I enjoyed it, feeling almost like a minstrel singing to my lover on a Venetian balcony.

Probably because we were paying more attention to each other, our lovemaking improved in frequency and quality. We enjoyed it more than we had for several years. Andrea had more strength and vitality. She was more demonstrative and passionate. The hope she had gained from her response to her treatments and the assertiveness that came from her self-empowerment were aphrodisiacs for both of us.

Chapter

14

J UNE'S trip to Wisconsin left only July before Andrea completed
her treatments under Dr. Robins's hyperthermia and chemotherapy
protocol.

She now loved Madison and the Midwest. The harsh winter setting
we had first observed, when our fear made everything seem colder, had
softened with summer and our own improving outlook. Sailboats
scudded along Lake Mendota where before there had been sheets of
ice. The college town and state capital had an easy, friendly bustle that
was repeated almost everywhere we went as we strolled the streets and
window-shopped. Ian and Andrea had developed a close rapport; he
admired the strides she had taken as a patient, and her original reverence for him had only deepened. We became social friends, and he and
his wife, Floriane, joined us as we sampled the casual, inexpensive
restaurants near the University of Wisconsin campus. The two doctors
had met in Europe when they both worked in cancer-targeted hyperthermia; d'Oliere since had moved from oncology to psychiatry.

The hyperthermia unit staff was also happy to see Andrea. She
laughed off the rigors of the treatment and welcomed it in a way that

somehow made everyone feel they were doing what they had entered medicine to do.

During July's final treatment, Andrea received an overdose of heparin, the anticoagulant routinely injected in her port in small doses to keep it clear. The overdose required a correction of her blood's coagulation factors, and while Robins's team was doing that it found an infection in her port.

Ports are handled frequently, so infection of a port, when it occurs, is no surprise. But it is no less severe for being common. Andrea's infection kept her in the hospital for a few days and took an additional two weeks of antibiotics to wipe out. The antibiotic dose came already prepared, in a plastic bottle that could be hooked onto her belt like a Walkman. There was no need for a cumbersome IV pole; air pressure between the outer bottle and the collapsible inner sack that contained the antibiotic substituted for gravity and made the dosage flow. This allowed her to receive the dosage even when we were on the move. I hooked the antibiotics up to her port every twelve hours, no matter if we were at home, at a restaurant, or in the car traveling to Amagansett and the beach house.

I continued to give her the monthly series of interferon and somatostatin shots. She welcomed them as she did the hyperthermia. I always winced when I injected her, but she embraced the fever for the feeling it gave her that something was happening inside her body to destroy the cancer.

August came. Her hyperthermia-chemotherapy regimen was over, and her monthly CT scan showed her liver clear, with no trace of cancer. The LDH level in her blood remained around 150.

It was good news, the best we could have hoped for. Indeed, Andrea so far had responded better than any other patient in the trial. But we resisted reacting too enthusiastically. Andrea was in remission, but that did not mean she was cured. The Mayo Clinic protocol also could have produced a remission, yet the patients treated with it invariably suffered a return of their cancer. Wanting to prevent this, and influenced by the fact that she had suffered few side effects in treatment, we asked for more.

"I know the protocol calls for seven treatments. But why not one or two additional, just to be sure?" I urged Ian in a phone call, with Andrea also on the line. "She's tolerating it well, without serious side effects."

"Sid and Andrea, I can't," he said. "The protocol is based on laboratory work that shows the course of seven treatments to be the most effective. Going beyond that, once the cancer is in remission, there's no additional benefit."

"But this is the first time you've treated a cancer like hers," I argued. "She's responded so well. Maybe this is the case where additional treatments would make a difference."

"It would violate the protocol," he said.

I didn't volunteer that we had been doing that for months with the interferon and somatostatin.

"There are other factors, too," he added. "She got too much heparin, and she got the port infection. It makes me think I'm pushing the envelope too far. I keep wondering when the next mistake is going to be made. You know, you two persuaded me that Andrea would be just another patient, but I can't forget who you are and where you come from. And I've always found that if you do things differently for a VIP patient, something goes wrong. Anything we do for our regular patients is the best we can do, and anything we do beyond that, we usually screw it up.

"We'd better stick to the original program."

A S Andrea emerged from the immediate threat of cancer, her mother succumbed. Helen had been sinking from the time her leukemia was diagnosed in February. She had been in Sloan-Kettering since then, her stints of treatment broken only by occasional weekends with Marsha and her family, with whom Michael was staying. Helen died in August.

Andrea's response mixed anger and grief. She had lived in the vain hope that her mother would someday change and offer her the validation and support she craved. With Helen's death, Andrea's lifelong craving would never be fulfilled.

"She's never going to be here for me," she said.

Her anger extended to her mother's years of life. Andrea saw her mother's death at seventy-five in the light of her own cancer and the fear that her remission would not last. "It's not fair," she said. "She got all those extra years. She got to be well until she was old, and I got cancer at forty-five. I'd give anything to have those thirty years."

We all went to the funeral together. Michael seemed broken without his wife. I felt for him, because I knew how alone I would be without Andrea.

W E had said we wanted to return to a normal life, a life before cancer. But things were almost better than they had ever been. The life we lived that summer of the antibiotics, and hyperthermia and chemotherapy, and interferon and somatostatin, the continued CT scans and blood tests, our meditations and walks together around the neighborhood, the performances we attended, even the mixed feelings that accompanied her mother's death, was more intense and vivid than the life we had known, the "normal" life we wanted to regain. Andrea's cancer had threatened to overwhelm us in so many ways. Yet it had created a spirit and focus that erased mundane, unimportant things and made each day a challenge to be mastered. And we had done it, Andrea most of all.

Would we have traded that for her not to have cancer? Of course we would. But the fact that we were paying a high price for the lessons we learned did not reduce their impact. Living as if death was just around the corner made each moment and each day more significant.

At the summer's end, we were almost always at Amagansett. It was our escape. We had built the house early in our marriage to replace a smaller one. Andrea had seen to the details, shaping it to fit our growing family, and she had always loved being there. It was close to the beach, high on a sand dune, with decks front and back, a pool, and a lot of glass so you could see the ocean whether you were inside or out. Andrea made good her pledge to devote time to the people she cared about. Her improvement gave us permission to invite good friends out on weekends, and with our Amagansett neighbors dropping in, the house was a center of activity.

We walked on the beach with Daisy every morning. The Yorkie was so small and light she skittered along the sand more like a bird than a dog. Andrea carried her when she got tired and couldn't keep up.

Andrea's concern over reinfecting her port kept her from swimming. She spent most of her time in her preferred spot on the deck, next to the pool under the shade of an umbrella, reading or watching the ocean, feeling the breeze that made the beach grass sway. I had the feeling, watching her, that she was trying to meditate on each moment as it passed, to capture it somehow in the feel of the air on her skin or the glint of light on the water. Afternoons lured me to the beach, where I would sit in a lounge chair and read, or talk with whoever happened to be with us that weekend, the kids and their friends, or ours. And invariably, there was a moment, caused by the angle of the sun or a shift in the breeze, when I would start to look for her. I would turn and not see her, and then I would turn again, and my heart would jump to see her coming off the road down the slope of the beach, wearing a straw hat that shaded her face and a long thin sundress and walking with a sinuous grace. She might be carrying some fruit for us to eat. Her arrival would change the conversation from politics and baseball to books and movies, or people and what they were doing, their feelings and thoughts, until the sun fell and the wind blew cool off the water.

The belief returned, for all we did to put it off, that time might, after all, go on forever.

THEN Jonathan announced he would not be returning to Columbia that fall.

"I'm going to take a year off," he said. Soon after that, he was on his way to California with a friend.

Andrea was shaken. She had always wanted to believe that attentive, caring parenthood produced attentive children. They would grow into adults who would enjoy their parents' company and want to spend time with them. It had troubled her, as the children grew older, that one day they would be independent of her. She wasn't sure what she would do when they needed her less, or not at all. Jonathan now seemed to be accelerating the moment of his independence.

Daniel continued to live at home, however. He still worked part-time for a colleague of mine at the Gastroenterology Service, while he continued his courses in the adult education curriculum at New York University.

Joanna started her senior year at the Bronx High School of Science. She was trying to find her autonomy in the way all teenagers do. She spent a lot of time with her friends, and when she was at home, she hibernated in her room with its own TV and phone. We didn't see a lot of her.

Andrea's remission had signaled the children that they were free to pay attention to themselves again.

I continued to give her the monthly series of shots the Atlanta doctor had prescribed, interferon in six-, eight-, and ten-million-unit doses, followed by somatostatin. She believed that they would help her immune system combat the cancer's return. There was nothing to say otherwise, and I was willing to meet her wishes, although it still made me wince to give her the shots. She continued on her regimen of vitamins and low-fat diet, her daily walks, and her three-day-a-week job at Dr. Sherman's office. Otherwise, we resembled the family we were before her cancer.

Jonathan returned in October and moved back into the apartment. Our closeness restored, all together in the same four walls, old family strains reappeared. One night, Jonathan and I both got home too late to appreciate the Chinese meal Andrea had gone to a lot of trouble to prepare. She and Joanna and Daniel had eaten together, but it wasn't the same when we got home, or if it was, we failed to say so. Jonathan, in addition, didn't feel like telling her where he had been.

"Nobody appreciates me," Andrea burst out, flinging her arms in a typically dramatic gesture. "Jesus, I'm the mother. Can't somebody appreciate me?"

I had learned in therapy long ago to step back at such times. Dr. Schmidt had said that feeling unappreciated was a problem related to her parents that Andrea needed to work out on her own. I retreated to the living room. Andrea ran into the bedroom. Daniel called her a crazy bitch and me an asshole, and Joanna and Jonathan both disappeared into their respective rooms.

Later Andrea and I made up and made love. She was describing all this to Schmidt at their next session, when the psychiatrist launched a harangue that shocked me in its blame-the-patient venom and made me wonder anew if he were not driving Andrea out of some need to project on her a fate he wanted for himself. My shock came later, when I listened to the tape that she brought home; Schmidt recorded all his sessions, and she sometimes asked him for a tape when she wanted to remember something.

She had been telling Schmidt about my initial reaction to her outburst. "He adores me when I'm happy," she said. "He likes me better when I'm cheerful. But the minute I feel bad, he has a tendency to fall apart."

"The minute you feel bad, you fall apart," Schmidt replied.

The answer stunned her. At least there was a long pause on the tape. When she spoke again, she argued that she was learning not to undermine herself.

"You remember the time I told you I was supposed to make restaurant reservations and waited too long and every place was booked, and you told me I wanted to be rejected? I've never done that again. I got over it. I use that. And last night, I got over my tantrum, and I could talk about it afterward with Sid and we had sex. It was wonderful. I feel very good about that."

In the next breath, however, she had returned to her life's great disappointment. "I wanted to act. I anticipated and felt I needed to study in the summer, and I went to the music and theater camp of Bard College. I majored in theater and minored in dance and got the lead in a play and studied all summer long. I felt I needed to be in a children's theater, and I studied at the American Academy of Dramatic Arts and at the Herbert Berghof Studio. That's when I told my mother I needed an agent, and that's when she really laughed. And that was the end of the agent. That was the end of a lot of things."

"I feel great danger," Schmidt said.

"Why?"

"Go on," he urged.

"It was the end of anticipating. But I had a plan. I knew what I wanted and I did it. I didn't get overwhelmed. I was able to try what I wanted."

"I feel great danger," Schmidt repeated.

"Danger that I'm not trying enough?" Clearly, Andrea had absorbed the message that she held the power to reverse her cancer.

"No. That despite all the effort you put into treating the cancer, treating the liver, getting the hyperthermia, getting the chemotherapy, getting the interferon, getting the somatostatin, all the beautiful recovery that you've undergone, all the work you've put into it, it will come to nothing because of the memories of your mother thwarting your effort to enter Performing Arts at the last minute after you had done all those things the right way. You did everything right, everything you were supposed to do. And then you failed because of your mother and your father."

Imitating her parents, he said, would lead her to sabotage her own recovery. "The problem is, you remember what your parents did, and say, 'This is what I deserve.' You will do everything right, with discipline, and forethought, and planning. And now comes the danger that you will remember how they thwarted you at the last minute."

Andrea protested, again, that she was learning. "We were able to avoid that at the hospital. When I was afraid I would die on the operating table and I postponed the surgery."

"That's chicken feed," Schmidt retorted. "That's a small problem compared to what we have to deal with. The urge is in your mind to imitate your mother and destroy your recovery at the last minute. Armageddon. That's what we are heading for. It's going to be your attempt at imitating your mother and father and denying you the benefits of your recovery at the last minute. Just like they denied you the benefit of all the work you put in going to Performing Arts. Because they were stupid, spiteful, hateful. And that's what you are going to do. I know it. I can see it coming. It will feel to you like your life depends on giving up the remission. The only way in which you can be loved and esteemed and valued by your parents is if you give up your recovery. It's going to feel to you like the right thing to do is to get sick and die."

"You're not saying I will do it."

"You'll feel compelled to do it. And you won't listen to me. My voice will disappear."

"Your voice was there last night," she said.

"But when this crisis comes, my voice will disappear." Schmidt berated Andrea for not listening to him. "I am talking into the void," he said. "You can't hear me, because your mother couldn't hear you and didn't listen. And rather than remember how painful it felt and get over it, you are just repeating what she did by reversing roles. I am Andrea, you are the mother, and you will ignore what I say.

"There are certain ways that you behave that are really idiotic," he persisted. "You have a tendency to be like Pollyanna, and when the sun shines for a day you think the world is wonderful. Bullshit!

"You had better think very hard and very profoundly about these things. Otherwise there is a calamity looming on the horizon."

The tape ran on, then out. I was horrified. I saw that Schmidt was trying, almost desperately, it seemed, to shift the blame to her parents, to force her by blaming them to give up her feelings of unworthiness. I understood his level of frustration. Andrea's years of therapy and the persistence of her anorexia showed a stubbornness. She seemed to cling to her pain, to cherish the hurt caused in her childhood, to not want to let it go. Like Schmidt, I wanted her to get it behind her. But to place the possibility of a recurrence on her shoulders still seemed irresponsible at best. Why should she, or any patient, carry such a burden? It fell into the trap of metaphor to attribute a pattern of behavior to a cancer, but her cancer's behavior meant it might very well recur. Schmidt was being too harsh, too quick to place blame for what, after all, was in all likelihood a random occurrence. I saw no Freudian shadows over her cancer, past or future, and I couldn't shake the thought that Schmidt had more at stake in her outcome than either Andrea or I knew.

JONATHAN stayed at home for a couple of months. Then he found a place of his own in the East Village, and another period of absentia began. He worked as a lifeguard at several health club swimming pools and also took room service orders at the Royalton Hotel on 44th Street. He wore earrings, grew a goatee, hung out with friends who were mostly older, and we didn't hear from him for weeks on end.

When we did, Andrea and I would ask how he was doing, what his apartment was like, who his friends were, if he was doing okay. He didn't like being questioned. Inevitably, we would argue, and another month or six weeks of silence would ensue.

I didn't know then why we fought. Jonathan later told us he thought of that time as his "little war of freedom."

Chapter

15

ANDREA'S remission continued. Freed from the immediate fear, we were tempted to resume life as usual. But we could not. Whatever happened next, we had endured a major, life-threatening event. Even if it never returned, her cancer would not pass from our lives without effect. We needed to take stock. We needed to look at our lives, absorb what we had learned about each other, and incorporate the lessons our new situation had provided.

The cancer's first lesson was a lesson in time.

Maybe we had years ahead, but maybe we had only months. Looking back at the months just past, how they had raced by and the new activities into which we had thrown ourselves, the intensity with which we had lived since Andrea got cancer seemed preferable to the way we had lived before. Then, days had passed by routinely, stretching into weeks and months, and while we lived fully, it seemed that we always were looking forward to high points down the road. Whatever time we had now, it seemed important to make more of it.

That required paying more attention. To everything. To each other, to the people around us, to the sights and sounds and textures of our lives. But to each other most of all. We started to just live in the present.

Scholars and experts suggest this attention to the present is one important step toward achieving wellness and an improved quality of life. Jon Kabat-Zinn calls it "mindfulness." Kabat-Zinn, the head of the Stress Reduction Clinic at the University of Massachusetts Medical Center, is an expert on meditation as a means of reducing stress and pain. In *Full Catastrophe Living,* his book that describes the clinic's program, he quotes an eighty-five-year-old Kentucky woman. "Oh, I've had my moments, and if I had to do it over again, I'd have more of them," said Nadine Stair. "In fact, I'd try to have nothing else. Just moments, one after another, instead of living so many years ahead of each day."

Bernie Siegel says the same thing in his new introduction to *Love, Medicine & Miracles.* Recounting his stories of exceptional cancer patients who defy the odds offered by conventional medicine, he says, "Remember, these people didn't set out to not die. They set out to live until they died.

"Please live as if you are going to die. Let your child out and enjoy the moment."

In that spirit, when Andrea talked, or one of the children, I listened harder and tried to hear better. I responded according to what they were saying, instead of to my own concerns. There was so much clutter to be pushed aside. But gradually, focused by the sense that time was not unlimited and urged to bring our issues to resolution, we discovered what had been there all along. Small things grew large, and the great, weighty issues shrank in proportion and became easier to handle.

I found joy in the smell of coffee in the morning. Andrea interrupted our conversations to point out a full moon. Together, we began to understand Jonathan's resistance to our questions. Our arguments, and the ensuing silence, were part of a war not of freedom, but of misunderstanding. He was unhappy, didn't know why, and when we asked how he was doing, he didn't like confronting his unhappiness. When he said, "Don't ask," we took it as a signal to back off, and he took our backing off as a lack of interest. But through time and effort, we learned how to relate to one another.

I THOUGHT a lot about Andrea's transformation. Schmidt saw her still mired in the past, but I had seen changes I hadn't thought possible. The level to which she had orchestrated her own course of treatment, and added components of her own from alternative medicine, continued to amaze me. This presented a dilemma. On the one hand, it solidified my belief that the patient's role in preventing and fighting disease was indispensable. I felt on the other hand that patients could assume too much responsibility. It was just as unreasonable for patients to take on the full burden of healing themselves as it was unconscionable for a doctor to blame a patient's personality for the disease. What was needed was a middle ground.

Andrea, I believed, had found this middle place, where hope had inspired her to adopt good habits, but had not led her down blind alleys away from conventional treatment.

I thought, too, about what I had learned about being a doctor since accepting my role as her spouse. Looking from the patient side, I realized that what I appreciated most from the doctors treating Andrea was their time. When she was entering the hyperthermia protocol, Ian Robins patiently explained its processes and possibilities, its pros and cons. Later, the doctor in Atlanta took the same care in describing what she could expect from interferon. This time spent in explanation did wonders to create a positive outlook that Andrea and I used to her advantage. I thought of my own schedule, which before Andrea's cancer had been crammed with the demands of administration and research, the lectures and medical meetings, on top of the time I spent with patients. Time was so precious, yet it was often what the patient needed most.

Andrea's respite allowed me to put some of this new knowledge into practice. My clinics began to run overtime as I took more time with patients, hearing them emotionally as well as medically. I was unable to move quickly from one patient to the next, because I was asking how spouses and children were handling things and jotting down suggestions for readings on meditation and stress reduction. I listened because now, being there myself, I knew what support really meant. Members of the clinic staff, instead of tapping their feet and looking at their watches, accepted my new approach as something quite natural. They were as excited as I was by the response shown by the patients.

One thirty-four-year-old woman came with her widowed mother. Ethel had cancer of the pancreas and the prognosis was not good. Her daughter was upset because Ethel had rejected her suggestions to take vitamins and meditate.

"What does she do to alleviate her stress?" I asked.

"She prays."

Ethel told me she was an observant Jew who prayed daily. I had grown up in an Orthodox Jewish household and continued as an adult to keep my connection to Judaism by going to temple and having traditional Shabbat dinners. Now, listening to Ethel explain the consolation she found in prayer and nowhere else, I realized I had found yet another resource.

"Prayer can be powerful, too," I told the daughter. "Maybe it's the most powerful thing of all. Prayer and meditation really are the same thing."

I suggested that she follow her mother's lead, and support it. The mother, in prayer, gained empowerment and a feeling of control.

"Step back. This is what she wants," I said. "Let her maintain her independence. Just be there for her and listen, and let her follow her own path. Just help her, and try to understand that you can't control what happens."

The daughter told me later how relieved she was to be free of the burden of her mother's outcome. She saw her role more clearly, and became truly helpful as she stopped trying to maintain control. Ethel, in turn, found a new bond with her daughter that enriched them both.

RECENTLY I came across a line in a novel that captures the essence of what patients want from doctors. In *The Ghost Road,* English novelist

Pat Barker has her narrator describe a healing massage given by a South Seas medicine man: "Once again that curious hypnotic effect, the sense of being totally focused on, totally cared for."

Andrea hadn't seen any medicine men. I knew, however, that the directions she had chosen might be viewed that way by some conventional doctors. The doctor in Atlanta, especially, would not fit criteria for working within conventional frameworks.

Empathy, the quality the novelist described — or call it bedside manner, if you will — is shared by many doctors, in conventional and alternative medicine and in traditional or nativist practices that give us medicine men and women. Empathy can be a powerful instrument. So powerful, in fact, that if patients don't detect it in one doctor, they may gravitate toward another they perceive as being more concerned about their healing. Conventional medicine's concern is that, in some cases, empathy can be misused to lure patients from proven treatments to false promises. It drives conventional doctors up the wall when patients reject treatments that may save them and go off in search of a will-o'-the-wisp. That's why much of alternative medicine gets a bad rap from the mainstream.

That was not the case with Andrea so far. She had pursued nonconventional therapies with unproven possibilities, but only in conjunction with treatments that fell within conventional norms. No one had tried to divert her from the mainstream. The hyperthermia, though experimental, was part of a rigorously monitored trial at a major medical institution. Bernie Siegel did not promote guided imagery as a substitute for chemotherapy. Larry LeShan did not tell her meditation alone would cure her. (We hadn't talked about the so-called cancer personality.) Even Dr. Schmidt and the man in Atlanta, while knowingly suggesting that she violate an accepted protocol, did not urge her to use interferon and vitamin supplements instead of hyperthermia and chemotherapy, but in addition to them. All of them, Siegel in his books, LeShan in his lectures, and the other two directly, tried only to enhance what conventional medicine was doing. Andrea took the best of their advice and built an integrated program.

Complementary or integrative medicine are better terms for what we were doing. Alternative medicine, as the word "alternative" implies, is considered a substitute for conventional medicine. Andrea chose enhancements, not substitutes. Complementary medicine combines science with a wide range of other knowledge to produce a whole greater than the sum of its parts. It recognizes that, along with great advances like vaccines, antibiotics, and chemotherapeutic agents, there is a wealth of experience as old as human history to be applied to the treatment and prevention of disease.

I had been skeptical at first. Now, my skepticism had been overcome by the results, and by Andrea's intelligent determination.

Dr. Schmidt, with his fondness for military metaphors, would have said that complementary medicine brings the complete arsenal to bear against cancer. An arsenal composed of the best weapons of modern science and tactics drawn from human wisdom and experience.

Andrea, in using complementary medicine, wasn't grasping desperately for straws. She was using bricks and mortar to build her house as strong as possible. She embraced the words of the nineteenth-century English philosopher John Stuart Mill, who wrote, "Over one's own body and mind, the individual is sovereign."

ANDREA'S remission was followed by partial remissions for several other patients in Ian Robins's trial. Andrea's result was all the more impressive because the CT scans showing her liver free of tumor were being done and interpreted at Sloan-Kettering. The trial's overall success was drawing renewed attention to the possibilities of hyperthermia. I wanted to help spread the news, and so I invited Ian to New York and Sloan-Kettering to lecture at Medical Grand Rounds.

When he arrived in November, Andrea and I met him at the airport.

The rapport between the two of them was undiminished by Andrea's completion of the trial. While Ian had declined to continue her treatments, he remained her oncology consultant. She called him to discuss each new blood test and CT scan result. During our dinners together in Madison, she also had forged a friendship with Robins's wife, Floriane. But perhaps she was closest of all with their young adopted son, a Tanzanian orphan named Amani, the Swahili word for peace.

Ian in turn was fascinated by Andrea as a patient. He was highly intelligent, endlessly curious, with multiple university degrees, including a Ph.D., and a certification in hypnosis. Andrea's willingness to meet her disease head-on is what intrigued him. Like many doctors who treat cancer, he had seen a fairly high percentage of patients fall into depression at their diagnosis. Yet Andrea had stayed upbeat. He knew something of her history in therapy, and he wondered what Dr. Schmidt had done to focus her.

"She told me that the stress of the disease, challenging her, had made a change in her life," he said. "What I want to know is, what happened?"

My interpretation was that Schmidt had gradually penetrated the layers of Andrea's personality and, to use an expression he favored, peeled them away one by one, like the layers of an onion. When her cancer was diagnosed, some of the subconscious layers that had made her passive and prevented her assertiveness from coming out already had been removed, and she was ready to respond. The cancer had simply accelerated her progress to assertiveness.

We spent the evening together at the theater. The play, *Dancing at Lughnasa,* might have been a metaphor for Andrea's experience with cancer. It was about the trials and disappointments, and the defiant, foot-stomping spirit, of a group of Irish peasant women. The spirit survived all their reverses, and shone through.

Dr. Schmidt, to my surprise, showed up for Ian's Grand Rounds presentation. He was wearing jeans and a sweatshirt, in contrast to his buttoned-down appearance in the office. I introduced him to Ian. They greeted each other warmly, and I was even more surprised to learn they knew each other.

Ian had entitled his talk "A New Focus for Cancer Therapeutics." He had been trumpeting hyperthermia's potential for years. Now, the results of Andrea's trial were bearing him out, and he argued passionately and persuasively that systemic hyperthermia should be considered as an adjunct for the treatment of cancer.

"How do you know Casper Schmidt?" I asked him when the talk was over. I had assumed that Schmidt had drawn his knowledge of hyperthermia, and of Ian's program at Wisconsin, from the vast medical encyclopedia he kept in his head and in the books and journals in his office. That they might actually know each other had never occurred to me before.

"He called me out of the blue one day," Ian said. "He introduced himself as a member of ACT UP gathering information about the possible applications of hyperthermia in AIDS. Later, after Andrea was in the trial, he called and said he wanted to come to look into the program. He came out, and we must have walked around Madison and talked all day. We've stayed in loose touch."

ACT UP was a name I knew vaguely. It was — and is — a group of ad hoc volunteers dedicated to ending the AIDS crisis. Once again, I wondered about Schmidt's connection to AIDS, and assumed he had such patients.

"We had another mutual connection," he added. "He asked me about a doctor who had done whole-body hyperthermia for AIDS and reported a good result. It turned out that I had served on a National Cancer Institute commission looking at this guy. He had the world thinking he had found a cure for AIDS, but the NCI questioned the documentation underlying his report. The institute wasn't sure the patient actually had AIDS."

"Where was this doctor?" I asked.

"In Atlanta."

"What was his name?" I asked, although I was sure I already knew the answer.

He named the doctor who had seen Andrea and prescribed her interferon. In the months since, she had stayed in close touch with him, as she had with Ian. She called Atlanta almost every week, seeking his advice on vitamin supplements and diet and his input on treatment options.

I knew he was at odds with the National Cancer Institute. He had told Andrea and me that he thought the NCI supported drug-intensive treatments that were too expensive for many patients with AIDS and AIDS-related cancer. He was crusading to find alternatives, and had experimented with hyperthermia. His patient, he claimed, was HIV-positive, had Kaposi's sarcoma, community-acquired pneumonia, and other manifestations of AIDS. The NCI commission disagreed with his diagnosis and issued a critical report. Robins had been among the signers.

My judgment was more sympathetic. Andrea was well covered by my insurance at the hospital. But I could see how it disturbed doctors to see their patients consumed not only by disease but by the cost of drugs. The AIDS epidemic had created a corps of activist doctors. They felt the urge on their patients' behalf to rush past the slow machinery of research, proof, and subsequent approval, and they felt their patients' bitterness at a disease that impoverished them financially as well as in body and spirit. I still believed in the conventional proofs, in well-documented research. I didn't know if the Atlanta doctor's documentation was up to snuff or not. In one way he was doing what a doctor is supposed to do, trying to find answers that can help his patients. I knew how those doctors felt, having urged Robins to keep Andrea in treatment beyond the prescribed protocol.

But undocumented claims lead patients in the wrong direction. They raise expectations and create unfulfilled hopes. They ultimately help nobody.

"Schmidt had been curious about his work when it got so much attention," Ian said. "But I think the commission's report made him less enthusiastic."

That was news to me.

Chapter

16

THE New Year, 1992, arrived.
Andrea and I returned to our opera singer friend's for New
Year's Eve. Riding uptown in a cab, I thought it was a miracle
that we were going. It was a miracle that we were even here. So much
had changed. I didn't make resolutions before, but now I did: I would
try to love my wife and children better, pay more attention, take more
time; I would try to grasp the simple moments that, before last year,
slipped by unnoticed. I saw my life with Andrea and the children in a
new light. Her cancer had shaken us awake.

We rang the bell and stood at the door holding hands. When our
hostess, Pat Kadvan, opened the door, the warmth of her home flooded
out and embraced us. "It's Andrea and Sid," she called back into the
room. Heads swiveled, faces lit in smiles to see us, and I felt such gratitude that tears sprang to my eyes. I had to turn away and dab with a
handkerchief before I could go in.

All evening, the lights seemed brighter and the friendship warmer.
At the night's close, we hugged more tightly, cherishing such friends.

The first day of the new year dawned uneventfully, and that, too,
seemed like a miracle. One year had passed since Andrea's first symp-

toms. By the end of the week, we had marked the anniversary of Andrea's swift diagnosis in January 1991 and those horrifying early days when I thought she had just months to live.

With the new year and these milestones came new hope. Schmidt's dire forecast had not materialized. We thought, with guarded optimism, that maybe we would beat this thing. We tiptoed toward the belief that we really could get past it.

Daniel, after living at home for the last year, found his own apartment fifty blocks away, in the East 30s. With Jonathan exploring his new environment in the East Village, and Joanna at school or with her friends a lot, our nest was almost empty once again. Andrea and I spent long winter evenings alone, lying nestled together as we listened to Brahms and Bach and the great operas of Mozart, Verdi, and Puccini. When we read, it was no longer abstracts of cancer trials. We continued to explore further meditations. We also began to read the Bible.

I forget whose idea it was. Maybe mine, because religion had been such a big part of my family's life when I was growing up, and I found such joy in the Sabbath prayers and in the services at my temple, Shaaray Tefila on Second Avenue at 79th Street, one of the oldest Jewish congregations in New York. Or maybe it was Andrea's, because while her parents had not given her a strong religious education, she attended temple with me and the kids, and was attracted to the power of the Bible stories. Neither of us, however, had read the Bible at home during the twenty-six years of our relationship.

When I opened the book in our living room for the first time, I felt a wave of nostalgia. Even at a glance, I saw passages that were familiar and comforting. I thought of Ethel, my pancreatic cancer patient, who had found comfort in prayer. Andrea urged me to read out loud, as she had urged me to read meditations. And quickly, we both were immersed in the Psalms, and the Proverbs, and the writings of the Prophets.

We loved the Song of Songs best of all. The beautiful love song of bride and groom to one another, of the anguish of separation and the joy of reunion, of a love as strong as death, expressed all the passion and devotion Andrea and I had rediscovered thinking our time together would be short. I found among the reveries one short passage that contained all my love for her, and all my hope for the outcome of our battle:

> *You are altogether beautiful, my love;*
> *there is no flaw in you.*

THERE was no detectable flaw. But while we allowed ourselves some optimism, we never stopped fearing the cancer's return.

Andrea continued to have monthly CT scans. They produced enormous stress. She would meditate alone before each one. During the procedure, which I would observe from a control room, I watched the face of Dr. Botet, the radiologist, for some sign of what he saw. Even when he reassured me, I looked beyond his words of assurance to the scan itself for any irregularity that would confirm my darkest fears.

The emotional impact of the blood testing was even worse, since it was done each week. I waited nervously for the LDH counts until they were posted from Sloan-Kettering's lab to the requesting doctor on our internal computer network. I could access them as easily as Bob Kurtz could, and it was torture until they were posted. I ran to my computer every fifteen minutes. Hoping for the best, I feared the worst. Different scenarios ran through my mind: the relief I would feel if it was still around 160 and how I would share Andrea's happiness when I gave her the good news; my anxiety if the number was slightly elevated, up to 175, say, and how I would try to reassure her; last, if the number was way up, the stark fear and grim knowledge that the war really wasn't over, that it had only paused.

The fear was as constant as the hope. It followed us like a black dream. Only time would free us of the fear, and we had not had enough time. At some undefined point in the future we would stop wondering. Until then, the questions would always be with us: When is it going to come back? How and when is it going to surface?

Bob finally laid down the law to both of us. He told me to stop checking the results, and assured Andrea that she could afford to get the tests less often. In most cases, they would have been; it was only because of my medical access they were being done every week. "You're driving yourselves crazy," he said. "We can cut down the frequency, and you and Sid both will have less to worry about."

We both, frankly, were relieved.

O N the day of Andrea's April CT scan, we were looking forward to a festive weekend. My sister Joyce's son Jeffrey was getting married. Watching Dr. Botet as he performed the scan, I saw him hesitate. Later, looking over the film of the scan, he studied a specific area and decided to perform a sonogram.

We waited nervously for the results of the latter test. Bob Kurtz came into my office to tell us that the sonogram had "cleared the area."

But Botet was uneasy and I knew it. Bob was uneasy, too. It was still too early. We still were within the cancer's window of opportunity. The fear sprang back to the edges of our consciousness, like predatory eyes looking from the darkness outside the campfire.

On Saturday morning, we packed to drive to New Jersey for the dinner and party preceding Sunday's wedding. All five of us were in good spirits as we rode through the Holland Tunnel. A sense of family unity pervaded us as it had not done for a long time; we felt easy and not in conflict with each other. Andrea, especially, enjoyed having everyone so close. She was laughing and animated as we emerged from the tunnel into daylight and picked up the New Jersey Turnpike. Down the road, where industry gave way to countryside, yellow splashes of forsythia showed that spring was coming.

More than an hour into the ninety-minute drive, I suddenly got an odd feeling and pulled to the side of the road.

"What's wrong?" Andrea said.

"I don't remember putting the hanging bag with our clothes into the car."

I got out with the turnpike traffic whizzing by and opened the trunk. The bag wasn't there. I climbed back into the driver's seat and said apologetically, "We'll have to go back."

Laughter changed to moody silence as we headed back to Manhattan. Our short, pleasant trip had turned into a marathon of traffic, tollbooths, and stoplights. I pulled at last into our apartment's parking garage and asked the attendants if they had seen the bag. No one remembered seeing it, and it wasn't in the area where the car had been parked. It wasn't upstairs in the apartment, either.

Finally, afraid we would miss the party, we packed another bag and headed back to New Jersey. We all were disconcerted. Andrea was the most upset because she had envisioned wearing a certain outfit and now was stuck with her second choice. But the inconvenience faded once we got where we were going and got into the spirit of the wedding.

We returned home on Sunday evening, and the bag showed up the next day. One of the attendants had found it, put it in the office for safekeeping, then had gone off duty without telling anyone. We had our clothes back. Aside from the wasted driving, everything was fine.

Andrea and I visited Dr. Schmidt together a couple of days later. In the habit of telling him the things that go on in our lives, we described this episode to him. I think I offered it as an example of my forgetfulness.

"We don't know why these things are happening," I said.

Schmidt pressed his fingers together and rested his chin on the fingertips. "Wasn't there a questionable CT scan lurking in the background?"

Andrea and I looked at each other and knew he was right. The thought chilled. Each of us suspected, in our hearts, that maybe things weren't so fine as the sonogram had persuaded us to believe.

T W O weeks passed. We didn't talk about our fears. I think we preferred not knowing, advancing our hopes to the next test while we let the suspicious CT scan slip into dim corners of our memory. I suppressed it, and Andrea did, too. May arrived, and she went in for her monthly blood test.

I was in the endoscopy unit, reviewing x-rays at a view box with Moshe Shike, when Bob Kurtz walked in. His voice, behind us, said, "The LDH is six eighty-nine."

For a second, I didn't realize what he was saying. It sounded as if he was talking about a test on another patient. Then I turned around.

Bob's face was grim, his eyes searched mine, hoping I would understand. "The LDH is six eighty-nine," he repeated. "We've got a problem."

I had dreaded this moment, but there was no way to be prepared for it. The scenarios I had envisioned when I checked the computer for her LDH were totally inadequate. I felt my face go hot and cold, and my heart plunged like a roller coaster before steadying. Andrea's LDH level, in remission, had been consistently around 160. April's test had shown the same level, indicating that her remission continued.

I followed Bob into his office. He sat down at his desk and called Andrea. He insisted that it was his role as her doctor. He got no argument from me. He wanted to discuss a plan of action so she wouldn't be left hanging with the bad news.

"Let's repeat the test," he told her. "It's been normal for months. Now it's so abruptly elevated, the first thing I want to do is make sure it's accurate."

Andrea practically flew to the hospital. She was there in fifteen minutes. She entered Bob's office shaken and in tears. "I can't believe it," she cried. "Everything has been so good. It was fine last month."

The nurse who drew her blood had trouble getting the needle in her port because she kept drawing deep, agitated breaths.

The repeat test was confirmatory, 710. There was no mistake. What Dr. Botet had suspected on the CT scan had been a harbinger; her cancer had come out of hiding and seemed to be on the march again.

We knew that it was possible, of course. The prior history of Andrea's cancer warned us that a recurrence was not only possible, but likely. The hyperthermia and chemotherapy had done their work, wiping out the vast majority of cancer cells. Presumably everything she had done — the interferon and the somatostatin, the vitamin supplements, stress reduction, all of it — had done some good. Schmidt, who had warned Andrea to be intensely vigilant, also had encouraged optimism by insisting, "You do not have cancer." It sounded good. It sounded right. We wanted with all our hearts to believe it. But a few cancer cells were clever and resisted destruction. They had lurked undetected for months, reproducing again and again until the numbers became large enough to be detected. Now they formed a reconstituted, reenergized army poised for another onslaught. We had been optimistic, but thought we would be prepared if this day came.

We were not prepared. We couldn't be, although we tried. Always some sunny corner of our brains excluded death, as it does for everyone until almost the last breath. I was as stunned as when I heard the initial diagnosis.

I recalled a dream I had as a child, a recurring nightmare from which I always woke with fear. At the time, my parents, my sisters, and I lived in a ground-floor apartment in a two-story house in Brooklyn. It was a long apartment, like a railroad flat, with a corridor leading from the front door to a dining room and kitchen, and then my bedroom and the bedroom my sisters shared in the back. In the front were the living room, my parents' bedroom set off by French doors, and a closed porch where we had a piano. In my dream, a lion was in my parents' room. I ran to close the French doors and then moved the piano bench against the doors and knelt on the bench, pushing against the doors to keep them closed. I was pushing and scared and suddenly I heard a growl behind me. I felt the lion's hot snarling breath on my bare bottom and I whirled around in fear to find it licking my ass as if getting a taste of the meal to come.

That is how I felt at Andrea's recurrence: vulnerable and mortal in spite of our efforts.

Human solutions had failed. Remembering my childhood dream, the only thing that gave me comfort was another memory triggered, it seemed, in several ways: by my patient who prayed; by the reading of the Bible that Andrea and I had been doing; by the thoughts of my own religious childhood. I remembered not just practicing religion, but surrendering to faith. Now I wanted to relocate the source of that faith and give myself over to the grace and generosity of God.

Chapter

17

As a man of science, I had strayed somewhat from my Orthodox upbringing. My father, Nathan, and my mother, Sally, came from the Ashkenazi tradition of Polish Judaism. They came to this country between the world wars, escaping the anti-Semitism of eastern Europe and finding religious freedom. I was raised with a strong belief in God. When I was five and my older sister died, my parents were crushed, but I saw the strength of their faith. Like Job, they wondered at life's purpose, but never believed that God had abandoned them.

They kept a kosher house. My parents, I, and my sisters sat down each Friday night to the ceremonial dinner that initiates the Jewish Sabbath. We lit candles, said prayers, sang songs, and ate good food. I learned at the Shabbat table of my family heritage. It included musicians, chess masters, doctors, Hebrew scholars, and composers of Hasidic music. The family attended temple together on Saturdays.

They switched me to a yeshiva when I was halfway through elementary school. There, in addition to my secular education in reading, writing, and arithmetic, I studied under a rabbi's direction the Bible and its commentaries, ancient Hebrew law and customs, and my Jewish religious heritage.

I brought my faith and love of the traditions into my marriage with Andrea. Every Jew is a creature of tradition, but somewhere along the way I found that Reform Judaism offered a blend of old and new that appealed to me. Daniel, Jonathan, and Joanna all attended Hebrew school. With Andrea's illness, I had stepped down from leadership positions at Temple Shaaray Tefila, but we continued attending services on Friday nights and the high holy days. We continued, too, our regular Shabbat dinners before or after Friday services, dinners like my parents had. Andrea laid the table with a white cloth and lit candles in the silver candlesticks that came down from my grandmother. As my father had done, I led the Kiddush chant over sweet Manishevitz kosher wine, and the blessing of the traditional, braided challah bread under its ritual cover of an embroidered napkin. Together we sang the Zemirot, the sabbath songs of joy and celebration for the day of rest.

Andrea's family had come further from the old religious ways than mine. She was not so steeped in the traditions. I had to teach her the Shabbat prayers and songs. She looked forward to the high holidays, but for her they were more about inviting people in and getting together with family than about worship and prayer. Nor did she make a beeline to temple on Friday nights like I did. When the kids were young and we all went to the beach house on weekends, Andrea would walk in the door when we got there and head straight to the piano while the kids and I scrambled to make temple. For a long time I couldn't dress for Shabbat services without hearing her play pieces from "Scenes from Childhood" by Schumann. But we believed in the same God. She supported my commitment to a Jewish upbringing for the kids and understood religion's role in my life.

The fundamental belief in God we shared before her sickness was a belief in an abstract creator, the architect of springtime and moonlight and the moments of happiness we chanced upon and created for ourselves in each other and our children. But true faith comes from a yearning to believe in more than what our senses tell us, that behind the evidence of our tangible world is a force with motive and intent.

Now, with the news of her relapse, I found I needed to draw closer to that force. I grasped for its purpose in the way that my parents had tried to understand my sister's death. We were reaching out, desperate for help, needing the therapeutic value of religious faith.

That faith has therapeutic benefits is beginning to be widely recognized in medicine today. I had seen it in my prayerful patient. I saw it now in my own need as a patient's spouse. The medical importance of religion has been documented over and over again.

"There is at work an integration of medicine with religion, of spirituality with medical practice, the twin guardians of healing through the ages." Those were the words of Dr. Dale Matthews, a Georgetown University School of Medicine professor, speaking at a 1995 conference called to explore "Spiritual Dimensions in Clinical Research." Three other national conferences were studying the spiritual aspects of health at about the same time. The meetings were reported in the *Journal of the American Medical Association.*

Jeffrey S. Levin, a Ph.D. professor of family and community medicine at Eastern Virginia Medical School, has studied the effects of religion where patients were fighting diseases, including heart disease, tuberculosis, and cancer. In twenty-six of twenty-seven studies, religion had a positive effect.

Andrea and I were not unusual. Prayer, spirituality, and religious belief are central to most lives. We were among the vast majority of Americans shown by polls to believe in God, of which a substantial number attend religious services regularly. We believed in prayer. We believed that God could help us, that we might even see a miracle, and in that we also fell in the majority.

Astute physicians for years have realized that they could marshal the spirituality of patients as an important tool for healing. But our need to believe came from outside the medical profession. Nor did Dr. Schmidt encourage it, despite its documented role in relieving depression and reducing stress. Ignoring a patient's religious side, or worse yet, fighting it, can even be detrimental, as I saw in Ethel's case.

Now that I was on the patient side, I saw that a faith central to everyday life can be strong medicine, a medicine of which we doctors should be more aware and encourage whenever possible.

O N E aspect of our faith was belief in a life after death.

It was quite easy for us to reach this belief against the backdrop of our faith and the sudden reappearance of the cancer. If Andrea and I were not allowed to complete our journey on this earth together, then it must continue elsewhere, on another plane. The bookstores were full of books that explored life after death and near-death experiences, and we started to read them. *Embraced by the Light,* by Betty Eadie, led the pack of best-sellers, but many of the stories of near-death experiences were similar.

One that struck me was recounted by a woman who had been extremely ill, maintained on a respirator and intravenous feeding, in intensive care. She had the sudden and distinct impression that her heart stopped, her breathing stopped, and she died. She felt that her spirit left her body and hovered overhead, looking down on her body and seeing her body lying there motionless, surrounded by doctors and nurses frantically trying to revive her. She saw a brilliant flash of light coming from a tunnel to which she seemed to be headed, and somewhere in this tunnel she saw arms outstretched to her from a kind of amorphous spirit. She recognized this as a guiding spirit attempting to help her in her transformation from life in a physical state to a spiritual afterlife. The spirit was not the shrouded, spectral figure of death carrying a scythe; it instilled comfort, not fear.

The woman recounted that she extended her hands, grasped the hand that was held out to her, and started floating through the tunnel when suddenly it all disappeared and she reentered her body. Her first memory of waking was a nurse leaning over saying, "I thought we had lost you."

This pattern — of a spiritual energy leaving the body, witnessing its death, then being helped by guiding spirits through a brilliant light to a higher, spiritual level — reappeared in everything we read.

Near-death and death are not the same, of course. Nobody can tell us what happens after death. Nevertheless, these near-death experiences gave us a basis for conceptualizing what might actually happen. They crystalized my long-held belief in an afterlife. They seemed so right, so orderly, so true to my concept of what happens when we die that I embraced them enthusiastically. Andrea did, too. We found comfort in feeling that no matter what happened we would one day be reunited, in a different state than the one in which we existed on this earth.

Andrea found special comfort in the concept of the guiding spirits. If she had to enter a new form of life, she wanted to feel a presence accompanying her.

I think that people facing death fear more than anything being alone. No one wants to die alone. No one wants to find herself alone on the other side, away from all her loved ones. Andrea's wish was one I think most people share — to maintain some connection with the earth they are leaving behind.

One night we had just opened our eyes after meditating when she said, "If I die, promise to talk to me," she said. "I'll hear you. Tell me about our children. Tell me about Shirley, and about Daisy. Tell me what you're doing. Find a companion. Don't be alone. I'll talk to you, too. Promise that you'll listen."

"You're not going to die. We're going to beat this," I argued desperately.

"But if I do, we have to keep this connection between us. If I do, I'm going to give up the world and everything we have now, and that will be painful. But I'll survive in some form. A spiritual form. You'll join me someday, I know you will, and then you'll bring me up-to-date on everything. Until then, promise to talk to me. I promise to talk to you. Promise to listen."

She looked forward, not to dying, but to our reunion. We made a pact. I took her hand. "I promise."

I felt the warmth of a special connection, a unison of hearts, our minds so entwined they would never part no matter what our physical or spiritual state.

This belief that we would be connected in an afterlife was not a signal of defeat. Rather, it was an avenue of promise. We had not abandoned medicine. We simply added faith. Religious faith meant that we could trust the outcome of whatever steps lay ahead of us, whether they led to cure or not.

Chapter

18

ANDREA turned forty-seven on May 6. Her latest CT scan had revealed new spots on her liver. The children had taken the news calmly, Joanna at home and Daniel and Jonathan in phone calls I made to invite them to a birthday dinner. There was none of the panic that greeted the initial diagnosis. By now we had a sense of being able to survive.

We met at Carmine's, a large, loud, family-style Italian restaurant on the Upper West Side. The atmosphere didn't allow for gloom. We sat around a big circular table and ordered pasta, chicken, and wine. I worked hard to keep the conversation light and make sure everyone was cheerful. Andrea delivered a reality check.

"So the cancer's back," she announced, silencing the table. She let the silence build to a dramatic pause while she looked at each of us in turn. "Well, I don't mind saying I'm very disappointed.

"I'm disappointed, and I know all of you are, too. I don't want to be disappointed again. I'm going to keep fighting. I want everybody's help. But I don't like being disappointed, and I don't want it to happen again." She raised her wine glass and swept her hand across the table as if she could dismiss the cancer with a wave.

"What can we do?" Joanna asked.

Andrea's tough posture melted. "Oh, God, just be my kids," she said.

In an instant they all surrounded her, pushing aside the heaping plates of food as they leaned over and hugged her and promised they would be there for her in her new struggle.

Afterward, when the plates had been removed and the wine glasses were almost empty, I held Andrea's hand on the tabletop. The kids looked around to see if anyone was watching. Parents aren't supposed to show their love in public.

But I was so proud of her. Her courage thrilled me. It helped me to get past my own disappointment to new reserves of determination. We had blasted this cancer out of the water once. We had to believe we could do it again. We were still in this world, not yet ready for an afterlife.

IAN Robins arrived in New York several days later. He had come for a scientific meeting, but he stopped in my office to look over Andrea's charts and the most recent CT scan.

"It's definitely a recurrence," he said. "She'll have to be treated, but we can't go back to hyperthermia again."

"Why not?"

"She won't respond a second time."

"Are you sure?" I knew that any treatment was likely to be less effective when repeated after a recurrence, but I had held out hope that hyperthermia, so effective in her initial course of treatment, would remain an option. "She had such a good response the first time, with hardly any side effects. Surely it's worth trying again."

Robins shook his head. "It's too much of a long shot, and there's no time. With this CT scan and her high LDH, we're looking at an aggressive tumor. We don't want to waste valuable time we might be spending with a more effective treatment."

"Hyperthermia was a long shot, too."

"I know it was, Sid," he said. "And it didn't win."

"It did win," I argued. "It produced a long remission, without much toxicity. It gave us fourteen good months."

"It won't happen again."

Ian was immovable. He, and everyone else on Andrea's official treatment team, thought it was now time to administer the Mayo Clinic protocol.

"What can I hope for with this?" she asked the night after Ian, Bob Kurtz, and Fry Casper announced their consensus. She already had decided to stop taking the interferon and somatostatin. She saw them as part of the first round of treatment. Now, with the recurrence, she wanted to move on.

"Hope for the best, I suppose," I said.

"Will it be good enough?"

"We'll make sure it is."

ANDREA tried to be brave as the first cycle of the new treatment approached. The chemotherapy would not be easy this time. She suffered few side effects from the carboplatin she had received with the hyperthermia. Cisplatin alone would cause her hair to fall out and produce more nausea. I could tell, as she resorted more frequently to meditation and at other times was distracted, that she was frightened. I hoped her old insecurities had not returned with the cancer.

Joanna turned eighteen in June. In fact, within less than two months we had three birthdays — Andrea's, Joanna's, and then Daniel's. For Joanna's, the five of us went back to Carmine's for dinner. Andrea ate well, a sign that the cancer's return had focused her. Later, Joanna and her brothers, along with some friends of hers, went to the roof of our building for an impromptu champagne party in the summer night. It was nice to see them easy together. They had always respected one another, had listened and cared, and considered one another's feelings.

Andrea watched them out the door and turned to me. "You know, we raised real people," she said. "We did a damn good job. These are real people." Her voice had the same fierce fondness with which she had always held the kids. They had come along rapidly, all three in the space of four years between 1970 and 1974; they had brought enormous changes to our life and caused me, for so many years a bachelor, to make some big adjustments. Suddenly we couldn't just take off, as we had on a skiing second honeymoon to Austria two months after we were married. But with them, Andrea found her vocation. Their Hebrew school was for me, but on her initiative they attended music lessons, had math and language tutoring, and all manner of enrichment.

"They are, aren't they." I shared her pride, and we gave each other a congratulatory hug.

For all her pride, it wasn't easy for her to see Joanna turn eighteen. Our daughter would be graduating from high school in two weeks. Before long, she would be off to college. Andrea knew that Joanna could make it without her. I don't think she knew if she could make it without Joanna. What would substitute in her life for the children's need for her, now that the youngest was passing into adulthood?

SCHMIDT told her it was the cancer that she needed in order to feel loved. She brought home a tape from another of their sessions. When I listened to it, much later, I was overcome again by the profound ambivalence for Schmidt that marked all of our relationship. Was he really as cruel as he sounded, or was he lashing her psyche in an attempt to motivate? Did the same thought lie behind what he said as when he coached her to believe she did not have cancer? There was no doubt that she already had begun a transformation for which his therapy, over years, prepared her. For all of the harshness in his voice and words, I believed he wanted her to get well as badly as I did.

Her voice was brittle as she entered his office the week after Joanna's birthday. She was approaching her hospitalization for chemotherapy and needed reassurance. "Do you think I look cute today?" she said. "I feel like I look cute."

He was silent and she continued. "I feel like I'm ready to embrace this treatment. I feel like I want to get this medicine. I'm going to be bald in three weeks. I'm going to be a redhead or a blonde. Actually, I'm going to be both! Why should I have to be one or the other? I should be both, shouldn't I? I told this to my wig lady, and she said, 'You got it, honey.'

"Everybody loves me. And you know what? I love myself. I look cute. I look puffy, like I had a tooth pulled or something, but I think I look cute."

Andrea talked for five minutes without Schmidt saying a word. Finally, I heard on the tape his chair creak. "You didn't think you were entitled to feel safe and well-fed. And you still don't," he said in his clipped accent. "You are pretending you have overcome your problems when you haven't. It doesn't work."

There was a stunned silence, as there had been in the earlier session when he broadsided her. If he was trying to focus her to give up her problems instead of struggling with them all the time, I didn't know why he had to pour cold water on her enthusiasm. Why couldn't he encourage her, push her by building her up instead of tearing her down? She wanted him to define her. That gave him awesome power over her, and I thought that often he abused it.

"Do you think I'm noplace further than I was?" she asked at last. "Am I still intractable and stubborn?"

"The only thing that has made any difference in your attitude so far has been the threat of being dead. Being loved is being at death's door. Which is why one episode of cancer was not enough. That's a sign of a person being profoundly intractable and stubborn beyond all belief."

"Am I still that way?"

"Do you want to bamboozle yourself? Why do you ask?"

"Because I'm scared."

"You should be scared. You're addicted to a crisis mentality."

"You think that now . . . ?"

Schmidt interrupted her. "It depends on you. The future depends on what you want and what you do. I don't listen to anything you say, only what you do. Now you are sitting with your fists clenched. A living image of your mother and your father. You don't give up your conflicts because that's what feels normal to you. And we have to pull that out of your mind somehow. Like a big radish. A horrible big radish. We have to get rid of it."

I could see it. Where Schmidt got the image I could not imagine. But the picture of Andrea's childhood conflicts hit home to me. I saw a radish with a tapered, tangled root, and that image melted into my own image of the cancer as something grasping and burrowing, struggling for a new grip in her body even as she struggled with new drugs to deny it.

On the tape, Andrea was crying. "I don't want to have to climb another mountain," she sniffed. "But I'm better. I know I am. I had this basic feeling that was a feeling of failure. It was with me without letup twenty-four hours a day. And it's lifting. It's lifting somewhat."

But Schmidt told her she had another mountain to climb. "At the beginning of the life of someone who later develops cancer is a bad relationship, in which one despairs of ever being able to be loved by somebody, usually a mother, or a father, or both. Then, that someone discovers something in life that makes up for it — she has children. She devotes herself to them, and this feeling goes away. Because they genuinely depend on her. And then they go away. Three of them go away. They were wrenched out of your gut. This is your reaction."

The tape hummed on with the sounds of traffic outside Schmidt's apartment windows. I pictured the trees in Riverside Park, green with new leaves. I could think of no scientific basis for his telling Andrea she needed cancer in order to feel loved, nor any therapeutic reason whatsoever.

Andrea's voice came up. "So the way I've been feeling about myself, and the relationship that Sid and I have been developing . . ."

"They are genuine achievements."

Thank God, he didn't feel the need to put her down entirely. Since the cancer we had strived for more intimacy, more immediacy, more attention to the moment. We had tried to rescue our relationship from the rut into which so many fall. We weren't bad together, we just had overlooked so many opportunities to make it good. Much of it had been my fault. My head had been in my work, dealing with its demands while thinking there always would be time for us to do the things we wanted. The cancer put a stop to that. With attention paid, seeking the value of the present, we had drawn closer.

But what still seemed brutal about Schmidt's approach was that he praised us as a couple, not Andrea alone.

"We have spent nine years together in psychotherapy," Schmidt continued. "I really care about you. The difficulty is for you caring about yourself. I think you deserve to care about yourself. The more scared you get, the more of the past you are willing to give up. But unless you're scared, you don't give up anything. Don't model your parents' behavior and not love yourself. The only possibility is for you to love yourself in the way that you deserve, and to treat yourself nicely. If you can mobilize your stubbornness to do things nicely for yourself, look where you'll be."

I ached for Andrea, preparing for a new battle with the cancer, trying simultaneously to resolve her inner conflicts. Each of us is a traveler carrying a rag bag of identity that contains scraps from our earliest moments. We are always sorting through them and trying to learn. Sometimes we make mistakes. Sometimes we're lucky. We always have to be brave. But as Schmidt returned, over and over, to his reductionist view of Andrea's problems and her cancer, I continued to think how indefensible it was to place the burden on the victim.

Andrea, on the tape, at the end of the session asked Schmidt to walk her out. "I want to call you. I feel like I may need to call you."

The psychiatrist pointed out that he sometimes saw patients all day long. "I will try to get back to you as soon as I can," he said loftily. "But there are limitations."

Chapter

19

A N D R E A started chemotherapy a few days later.
The regimen combining cisplatin and VP-16 brought together a cancer killer and a cancer inhibitor. Cisplatin was the powerful toxin that would kill the cells; VP-16, or etoposide, was the inhibitor. It is a plant alkaloid also called epipodophylotoxin, which interferes with cell division. Data from other diseases suggested that repeated exposures were more effective than single exposures, so patients received VP-16 over three days. Cisplatin, with its tendency to damage the kidneys, had to be given with a lot of intravenous fluid to flush them. The combination added up to a hospital stay.

Andrea checked into Sloan-Kettering. We were familiar by now with the admissions procedure. It was like checking into a hotel. "Welcome to Club Nausea," she cracked.

Drugs dripped into her for the next three days, from bags suspended on an IV pole through a tube into the port in her chest. She received the VP-16 constantly and the cisplatin on the first and third days.

I sat with her. Sometimes, at night when she slept under sedation for the nausea, I lost myself in staring at the bubbles rising through the IV tube, air displaced by the descending liquid, ticking away, moment by moment. She slept a lot. When she was awake, she sat up and tried to will the nausea away.

The chemo, attacking normal as well as cancer cells, exhausted her. It drained her body's energy. Home again after the course of chemo was complete, she was knocked out for two days. On the morning of the third day, she dragged herself out of bed and went to work at Dr. Sherman's office. She was revived when she came home. Slowly, she returned to her daily walks, her cooking, her psychotherapy with Dr. Schmidt. Nothing kept her down for very long.

But chemotherapy's effects are like falling dominoes. First came the nausea, then the fatigue. Finally, and most dangerous, she faced the potential for anemia, bleeding, and infection.

A week to ten days after the last drop of chemo had dripped through her port, Andrea's circulating blood was a river of dead cells: white cells, which fight infection; red cells, which prevent anemia; and platelets, the keys to coagulation and the prevention of bleeding. The bone marrow that manufactured her blood's precursor cells also had been bombed out, and so it could not immediately replace them. Transfusions could put red cells back into circulation, and platelets also could be administered. Her bone marrow, however, was the only source of white cells.

To speed this vital source back to productivity, I gave her nightly injections of Neupogen. This drug, scientifically known as GCSF, or granulocyte-colony stimulating factor, was originally isolated in a Sloan-Kettering laboratory. It stimulates the stem cells in the marrow to produce white cells by chemically whipping them into action.

BY June 19, the danger of infection was over. Andrea and I, with Joanna and our neighbor Lillian Clyde, drove across town to the Jacob Javits Convention Center for Joanna's high school graduation. Mrs. Clyde was a fiercely independent widow who walked a mile every day and kept an encyclopedic knowledge of our family's birthdays and special events in her razor-sharp brain. She had no children of her own, so she doted on Joanna, Jonathan, and Daniel as a kind of surrogate grandmother. Andrea included her often at dinners and other family occasions. Mrs. Clyde had been to all of our children's graduations.

A cold wind off the Hudson River blew rain in our faces as we walked among crowds of students and parents from a parking lot to the convention center. We met Daniel and Jonathan in the lobby, and found seats in the auditorium while Joanna put on her cap and gown and joined her Bronx High School of Science classmates.

"It's hard to believe she's almost gone," Andrea said as we waited.

"You'll miss her, won't you? I will." Joanna was taking a summer trip to Europe and would start at the University of Wisconsin at Madison in the fall. Her choice of Wisconsin was coincidental. She had applied before Andrea's cancer was discovered and we started going to Madison for hyperthermia.

Andrea bit her lip and squeezed my hand. "They'll all be gone."

Daniel and Jonathan embarrassed Joanna by chanting her name as she walked onstage for her diploma. I thought in a flash about their childhoods, all so different from my own. Manhattan was "the city" when I was a boy, playing stoop ball and johnny-on-the-horse with my friends on our Brooklyn streets of two-family houses with driveways and backyards. It was a mysterious, faraway, and fascinating place where the boys all grew up to be like Jimmy Cagney. I tended tomato plants that never seemed to grow and listened to Texaco's Saturday afternoon opera broadcasts on the radio. We had block parties, and we poured into the streets to celebrate the end of World War II; my children watched the fall of the Berlin Wall on television. I spent my summers selling ice cream on the beach at Coney Island, going from door-to-door in the neighborhood selling magazines, and later babysitting; Daniel, Jonathan, and Joanna all went to summer camp. The fresh bread my father brought home each morning after his night shift at the bakery perfumed my boyhood kitchen; our apartment kitchen more often smelled of Chinese takeout.

But there were similarities as well. My mother, like Andrea, had put her children through piano lessons and other courses of improvement

with an ever-changing cast of teachers. And I, like my father, was too often absented by work. I thought of the times I had hungered for his
company, but he was sleeping and not to be disturbed, and then, at
night, he was at the bakery. How many days had I driven our children
to school in the morning and then not come home at night before they
were asleep?

Like Andrea, I was proud of our kids, and proud they had grown up
in Manhattan. The truth was, their childhoods were not nearly as exotic
as I imagined Manhattan childhoods would be when I looked at the island from afar.

Joanna took her diploma and stepped across the stage. I hugged Andrea around the shoulder and blinked back sentimental tears.

ANOTHER week, and Andrea stood in front of the mirror, dismay on
her face. She pulled a clump of hair out of her comb and turned to me.
"Look at this," she said.

I nodded.

She turned back to the mirror and ran the comb through her hair.
Each pass brought out new clumps. For a few days, there was hair everywhere, in the shower drain, on the sheets and pillowcases. Then she was
bald. There was no hair anywhere on her body. Her arms glistened
without their down of hair. Even her eyebrows and eyelashes were gone.

Her baldness astonished and attracted me. Hair is an adornment.
Even in an age of shaven sports stars and rock musicians, it's rare to see
what it conceals. Now Andrea's scalp was exposed, as naked and smooth
as innocence itself. I saw her as a different person. Her features, delicate
and beautiful, appeared as I had never seen them before. Suddenly her
ears were finer, her eyes larger and more exotic, her nose more sculp-
tured. I saw her more clearly, and I loved what I saw. I began to love her
more, if that was possible. Her physical transformation, coupled with her
emotional and personal strides, brought strong passions to the surface.

At night in bed, I caressed her head and kissed the smooth, tight
skin and told her how beautiful she was. "I didn't see how beautiful your

eyes were until you didn't have eyebrows," I said. "I never saw your ears before, they were always covered up, but they're so delicate. You're more beautiful than I imagined. It's like I'm seeing everything for the first time."

Her naked eyebrows lifted and her laugh came from deep in her throat. "Sidney Jerome, you're full of it," she said.

But she responded to my schoolboy ardor. It gave us a way to remain kids at heart, to cling to the optimism of our youth. We reimagined our lives by being playful and romantic. And I know it reassured her to know she was still attractive to me, as I was comforted when she ignored my first gray hairs. I had told Andrea on every birthday and anniversary that I loved her more than the year before, and it was always true. Now, it was doubly important to us both, not only to declare our love but to nurture and deepen it.

Andrea took baldness in stride. She accepted it as a sign of treatment and response, as she did the effects of hyperthermia and the fevers the interferon had given her. It meant her cancer was being attacked. If baldness was the cost, she would pay gladly.

A friend of Andrea's, her "wig lady," gave her her first wig. This friend had received chemotherapy for breast cancer. She had a response and was in remission. Andrea felt the wig brought her friend good luck and would do the same for her.

One wig was not enough, however. As she had told Dr. Schmidt, she wanted to be a redhead and a blonde, and why shouldn't she be both. "You can't just shampoo your wig and wear it like you can your hair," she told me. "I need two, at least."

Shopping for wigs became our game that summer.

We shopped at Theresa's wig shop on 60th Street between Second and Third Avenues. Theresa's not only was one of New York's biggest wig emporiums, it was fairly close to Sloan-Kettering and dealt with many chemotherapy patients. We would look over the selection in the window while Andrea decided if she liked blonde or brunette, curly or straight that day. Then we would stride in like oil barons invading Tiffany's. I would find a chair, and a show would unfold as Andrea gathered a selection of wigs and modeled them. She became Andrea the diva, Andrea the ballerina, Audrey Hepburn, Jackie Kennedy, Emma Thompson, Lauren Bacall, laughing and vamping as she acted out the personalities the different wigs gave her. She had a great time, and I saw the actress she might have been. I laughed with her, and offered my thumbs-up or thumbs-down vote on each selection.

It wasn't long before she had several wigs for almost every occasion or shade of personality. We were walking into a neighborhood restaurant one rainy night when she turned to me, in a black wig and trench-coat, and whispered in her smokiest voice, "So this is the most famous gin mill in Casablanca. My name is Ilsa. Go ask Sam at the piano to play it again. You'll do that for me, won't you, Rick?"

We both burst into silly laughter, and dined with a shared secret as delicious as the meal.

The wigs were hot, and she didn't wear them all the time. When we were at the beach house on weekends, and for the daily power walks that she resumed as the chemotherapy wore off, she preferred a baseball cap. Her caps were as jaunty as the wigs, but sometimes, usually when we were in public, her baldness struck me in a different way. It brought back the reality — it shouted cancer and tore my heart with its reminder of the brave battle she was fighting.

Chapter

20

F OR the several days after chemotherapy, when it was impossible
for her to exercise or go to work, she lay on the sofa in the living
room and read the Bible. I was seeing fewer patients again since
her relapse, so I would come home early from the hospital on those
days, and then she would ask me to read to her.

We had been reading the Bible for several months now. With the cancer's recurrence, she was finding different subject matter that appealed to
her. Before, we had read exclusively in the Old Testament. She still liked
the poetic resonance and beauty of the Song of Songs, and she still sought
to grasp the source of Job's patience in the face of the agony and torture for
which he had been singled out by God. But now she also wanted to hear
the Gospels of Matthew, Mark, Luke, and John in the New Testament.
She wanted to hear over and over again about Jesus, his trials and tribula-
tions and his questioning of God's purpose while he was on the cross.

"I can relate to that," she said of Jesus' question, "My God, my God,
why have you forsaken me?" "Why me? What did I do?"

She wasn't comparing herself to Jesus. But she felt she could relate to
Job's challenge of God's reasons for singling him out for disaster, and to
Jesus' feeling of abandonment. She was trying to understand how Job

and later Jesus responded to the tests they faced, how they handled challenges. The passages she favored conveyed the patience of love and the universality of suffering. She saw in Job's restoration and Jesus' transformation her own potential outcomes: she would get well, or find existence in another life.

Those were the questions she had when she was debilitated by nausea and the fatigue of chemotherapy. We read the Bible the rest of the time, too, returning frequently to the love poetry in the Song of Songs.

Here, both of us wanted real poetry, but we found at some point that the power of the language in my old Bible failed to match the power of the message. We wanted a poetry of words as well as thought, the kind of literary beauty we had found when I read to her from Shakespeare's *Sonnets* years before. We went Bible shopping. We browsed through old bookstores, poked in the back shelves for old Bibles that might contain what we were looking for. Finally we came across a worn but readable Bates edition of the King James version, an edition first published in 1936. We turned to what had become our benchmark passage, the Bride's Reverie from the Song of Songs, and found our poetry:

> *My beloved spoke, and said unto me,*
> > *Rise up, my love, my fair one, and come away.*
> > *For lo, the winter is past,*
> > *the rain is over and gone,*
> > *the flowers appear on the earth;*
> > *the time of the singing of birds is come,*
> > *and the voice of the turtle is heard in our land.*
> *The fig tree ripeneth her green figs,*
> > *and the vines are in blossom,*
> > *they give forth their fragrance.*
> *Arise, my love, my fair one, and come away.*
> *O my dove, that art in the clefts of the rock,*
> > *in the covert of the steep place,*
> *let me see thy countenance, let me hear thy voice,*
> > *for sweet is thy voice,*
> > *and thy countenance is comely.*

The message of love, of carefree days gone by, evoked deep feelings between us. The language felt timeless rather than archaic; it gave the love that was expressed a permanence. It fixed the love between husband and bride as my love for Andrea was fixed. It made me weep to read it, then and now.

As we read the Bible, we found a reverence that brought us to prayer. We prayed at temple and at our Shabbat dinners, of course, but this was different. Praying in a group, out loud, was a fixed, traditional ritual. I knew most of the prayers by heart, and their very familiarity soothed me.

We pray on the high holidays for forgiveness and that our prayers be heard. We pray for health and life for ourselves, our loved ones, and for all mankind. We give thanks for being permitted to reach this day. We pray that the sick get well. In all this praying it is understood that we must find our own strength and shape our own destiny, and that we cannot wait or expect the divine hand to work miracles for us. Days of atonement intervene, during which we are expected to put in place the changes for which we've prayed.

One prays silently at temple, too. But praying silently, alone with Andrea, was more comforting than I would have thought possible before our need brought us to the act. As I had told my patient Ethel's daughter, it was a form of meditation, but it was different. The appeal of praying was exactly what I remembered from my childhood. It was an act of surrender, of giving up authority, of admitting you can't do it all yourself. This was the opposite of the activism that doctors are used to. We always think we can solve the problem, but sometimes we can't. Praying was a way of holding in balance the wish to heal and the need to admit that sometimes things are out of our hands.

I never knew what Andrea prayed for when we bowed our heads together. She didn't tell me. I think it was like telling what you wish for; if you express the wish, it won't come true. I prayed to grasp the merest coattail of divinity. By that I mean, if I pictured myself in a long tunnel, I didn't pray to be at the end. I asked God to give me tools in the form of understanding, patience, courage, wisdom, so I might get there by myself.

It might have gone something like this:

"Dear God, ruler of the universe, please smile upon us and be gracious to us. Forgive our sins. Help us to understand the nature of your plan for us. Help us to see your way. Give us the patience to wait for it to become more clear. And if we cannot see your way, God, then give us the wisdom to know it is your way, and not ours. Give us the courage to face what you have in store for us. Help us to abide by your plan, whatever it is. If we suffer, help us to know that it is not our sins that cause it, but a passage in your plan. If we are to find joy, help us to appreciate it. Help us to find the capacity to laugh, especially at ourselves and our pretensions. Help us to appreciate and love each other, and to recognize even in the face of her disease your gifts to us — each other, our children, our friends, the good that we can do for others. Give us, please, these small gifts. Amen."

Sometimes I couldn't resist adding a postscript: "And God, if you just happen to be saving a miracle for someone . . ."

Did God hear me? Does God have the inclination to act on anyone's behalf? And by praying, were we better off than people who did not pray? Was Andrea more likely to be cured?

The key to those questions lies in the individual. I had been led through years of adherence to my faith to believe that the force that is God could be influenced on my behalf by prayer and by good deeds. Prayer, for us together, was an antidote to despair and an attempt at understanding. The solace I found in surrendering part of my burden to God, and the solace I'm sure Andrea found in her prayers, gave us a new fortitude. The understanding I gained by praying not for a destination, but for a map and a flashlight that would help me get there, strengthened me by helping me realize my needs. It was this fortitude, this feeling that we could go on, that medicine is starting to recognize as the healing power of religious values.

But faith, and lives that are spiritually attuned, that are generous and caring and respond to the sense that we are not alone, don't have to exist within a specific religious framework. What is most important is a source of strength, wherever it is found.

Andrea and I both received from our prayers at home an effect much like that produced by meditation. A certain calm descended over both of us, but it was more general than meditation gave us. Meditation got us through the night, or through the moment. Prayer and reading the Bible gave us a more lasting peace that came from increased hope and greater acceptance. We understood that, for us, there was a greater power and meaning in the universe, and that the ways of God truly are mysterious.

ANY response to the new chemotherapy would have been the small miracle I hardly dared to pray for. Andrea's resistant cancer cells had survived the similar platinum-based drug carboplatin. But she did respond. As the summer advanced, the telltale blood tests showed her LDH dropping from its frightening high. Her CT scans showed the spots on her liver getting smaller again.

As she improved, Ian Robins agonized that maybe, after all, he should have continued her on hyperthermia.

"When she relapsed, you would think that the disease would then be insensitive to the drug," he said. "Responding a second time probably meant we should have continued giving the treatments. I think it would have put her into a longer remission and — I can't say this medically — maybe even cured her. With two or three more cycles, she would have had a longer disease-free interval and, who knows . . . ? If I had a crystal ball."

He illustrated his thinking by describing a tumor shrunk to one centimeter by the time of remission, and ascribing to it 500 million cells. Each successive treatment would knock two zeros from the number. Oncologists say "two logs killed," as if the zeros are pieces of cordwood. Thus the cancerous cells would decrease from 100 million to 10 million, to 100,000, to 1,000. "And then, who knows?" he repeated.

If that were all there was to it, cancer treatment would be easy, and Ian knew that, too. There would have been risks in continuing the treatments. "Each time you give a new cycle, you can get people into trouble," he added. The treatments had their own drawbacks: stresses on the system, attacks on healthy cells, dangers like the overdose of heparin and the sepsis, the blood infection, Andrea experienced.

Furthermore, cancer cells don't always cooperate and die like chopped logs.

There was nothing to gain by looking back. I had tried to persuade Ian to continue the treatments, but he had had good reasons for declining. Andrea and I had to resist second-guessing and thinking about what might have been, and instead move forward.

Ian, in any case, had a backup plan. It did not rely entirely on chemotherapy.

THE year before, when the cancer was retreating, he had suggested that we prepare another option. "A bone marrow transplant will give us another possibility in case we need it," he said. "I'd like to put some of her bone marrow away when she's in remission."

In the fall, when the signs of the cancer had disappeared and Andrea's remission was complete, she had entered Sloan-Kettering's Surgical Day Hospital and, in a procedure that required only a few hours and light sedation, had bone marrow suctioned from her hip bones.

Bone marrow looks like and has the consistency of thick blood. It produces blood's essential elements — red cells that carry oxygen, white cells that fight infection, and platelets that stop bleeding by forming clots. Suctioned out in anticipation of a transplant, it is placed in sterile tubes so as not to become infected. Microscopic examination assures that there are sufficient numbers of "stem" cells to reconstitute the marrow and allow it to begin producing the necessary blood cells. It is then frozen with preserving agents, awaiting reinfusion into the patient after a massive dose of chemotherapy that will wipe out the existing marrow, and — as we hoped in Andrea's case — the cancer cells.

Fry Casper was administering Andrea's chemotherapy. Like Robins, he was surprised at how well she was responding. He expected the tumor spots in her liver to shrink and stabilize, not to disappear. But as signs of the cancer steadily diminished and Ian started pushing for the marrow transplant, Fry questioned the plan.

"You do bone marrow transplants when you're treating leukemias and lymphomas," he argued. These cancers involve the bone marrow as the source of the abnormal cells that are reproducing in the bloodstream or the lymphatic system. The point of transplantation — using marrow taken from a patient during remission or from an immunologically matched donor — is to destroy and then replace the abnormal cell factory. Andrea's cancer did not arise in the marrow. Marrow transplantation had not been used successfully for solid tumors like Andrea's and had never been tried with her specific type of tumor.

But Ian argued that a transplant would allow her to get the largest possible dose of chemotherapy in order to try to wipe out the cancer, without worrying about its effect on the marrow and blood cell production. It was this extra dose of chemo, a dose that mimicked the delivery effects of hyperthermia, that he hoped would wipe out the tumor.

"I can't deny that it might just work, if she goes into remission. But it's extremely risky," Fry persisted. "Five percent of patients die from infections. Are you prepared to take the risk?"

He was right, we were walking into extremely dangerous territory. Killing the bone marrow and wiping out white blood cell production leaves the body without resistance to infection. So infections are a constant threat, and five percent of patients do die from the complications of infection. The procedure is extremely expensive as well, making it off-limits for most patients without insurance.

Andrea talked to Dr. Schmidt and called the doctor in Atlanta for his view. "I don't think it's the solution, but if it's what you want, God bless," he said.

When the arguments all were made, Andrea said she wanted to go ahead if she reached remission.

THE summer lengthened. Andrea took up drawing. She attended classes, and one day I came home to find her sitting with a sketch pad in the living room, drawing a naked female torso. She ignored me when I looked over her shoulder. Elsewhere on the page were gracefully extended limbs and bodies in motion.

She finished shading the torso and looked up. She seemed as peaceful as she did after meditating. "I didn't know you could draw," I said.

"I could always draw, I just never did," she said. "I always told myself I'd start someday. I decided if I didn't start soon, I might never."

She quickly filled her first sketchbook and started another. She drew obsessively, as she once had practiced the piano. Her subject was always the same: the perfect female body. The bodies she drew were exquisitely muscled, the arms and hands slender and fine. Always, when she drew, she was focused and absorbed; nothing disturbed her.

I started framing her drawings, and hanging them in the den, but she drew faster than I could put them up. She was projecting her advancing remission, and her hopes for beating the cancer after all, onto the drawing page.

One Sunday she held up one of the newspaper travel sections. "Sid, look at this," she said.

I looked at a photograph of pastel houses descending a hillside to blue waters. The story was about Positano, a resort town on the southwestern coast of Italy.

"Let's go there," she said.

Chapter

21

I IGNORED Bob Kurtz's warnings and checked Andrea's LDH levels more compulsively than ever. Since the recurrence, she was having blood drawn once a week again, and I knew just when to start checking the computer for results. It marched steadily downward, each drop toward her normal level of 160 taking her closer to remission.

Meanwhile, Andrea fixed on Positano. I agreed to go, and we made plans. The town in the picture rose on her horizon and moved closer day by day. She woke up each morning with daily goals as well. She kept me guessing. One day she would decide to try a new recipe, the next, to complete a drawing.

Positano was a bigger goal. She held on to that picture from the paper and that image, as the chemotherapy pushed her toward remission. Positano was the bonus she was going to give herself at the end of the chemo, before the dangers of the bone marrow transplant. It was something to look forward to, along with seeing Joanna off to college.

Her push toward both short- and long-term goals reminded me of behavior I had seen in my patients. Many had told me of approaching birthdays or anniversaries, a child's wedding or a graduation, as if asking my permission to attend. A man with colon cancer wanted to know if he should travel cross-country to watch his grandson compete in a marathon. He was sick, but I said, "Sure. Go and have a great time. I'll see you when you get back."

I always gave my patients such permission. It was as good as any medicine. Hearing that it was okay to attend important, often faraway, events was an important message to the patients for whom these events were goals. They became confident that they could handle the situation medically and that they would survive through the event. Most of the time, they returned in better shape than when they left. They wanted to stay well until the occasion, and having that to look forward to helped them maintain a focus on being well.

Now that I saw Andrea setting goals and working toward them, I realized how vitally important pursuing both short- and long-term goals is to patients facing lethal illnesses. I saw that it would be worthwhile not just to respond to a patient's wishes to have his goals legitimized, but to encourage a patient toward goal setting.

And for Andrea, a week of peace and serenity in beautiful surroundings would help her gather strength and determination for the transplant. It would be a retreat before the next big battle. For the two of us, it would mean, for a change, not waiting for time to come to us, but grasping it.

ANOTHER problem intruded as that summer neared an end. My prostate gland had enlarged to the point where at times it was almost impossible to urinate. Many men in or past middle age will know the feeling. Mine was not cancerous. I was considering surgery to have it corrected, which, I was assured, would leave me neither incontinent nor impotent.

But events were piling up. Andrea was just coming out of the hospital from a course of chemotherapy, and Joanna was returning from Europe before packing for college. I could not make up my mind whether to proceed with the surgery, or to wait until everyone else was settled. Meanwhile, I was getting more uncomfortable day by day.

I agonized and finally took my dilemma to Dr. Schmidt. I told him I didn't know why I should defer my own medical care, but still felt compelled to wait. "I need your help in sorting all this out," I said.

I was looking for a sounding board, not a decision, but the psychiatrist sought answers deep in the subconscious. "It sounds like there's a spasm, and we have to ask if there's a psychological origin for it."

I didn't know what he was getting at. The origin was that my prostate was too damn big. I had recently spent a few days with a catheter. It eliminated the discomfort of constantly feeling I had to urinate, but it was no fun, either. "My feeling now is to wait," I told him. "But when I'm uncomfortable, I think, 'Screw everybody. I've got to take care of myself.'"

"It's not either-or," he said. "It's not them versus you. Everybody should be taken care of. In your mind there is the persistence of this idea that you are supposed to be everything for everyone, and that that excludes you. And the only way you can do that is by being stoic, by not dealing with your feelings. Holding your feelings. This sounds just like urinary retention. I think you were angry with Andrea, and this got dammed up, just like the urine. I don't think it's a coincidence that your prostate problems have gotten so much worse since the recurrence of her cancer. I think there are a lot of unexpressed feelings."

I wondered if it could be true, and realized that it was. It's hard to have the right and generous response to problems that affect your life, no matter how badly someone else's is affected. I suppose I had gotten used to Andrea's being well, and resented the impact of her being sick again.

"I am angry with her," I confessed. "I'm angry with her for all this ill health she's had for so many years."

"Have you told her?"

"No."

"How come?"

"All this anorexia she's had for years and years and years. Coming to see you so many times." Andrea had continued to eat better since the onset of her cancer, but at some level the anorexia persisted and she still fought to consume all the calories she needed.

"You're holding back on your true and genuine feelings."

"What am I going to say to Andrea, that I'm angry with her because she's been anorexic for so many years?"

"It's what you genuinely feel."

"It's a hell of a thing to tell somebody when she's facing treatment for cancer."

"She knows it anyway," Dr. Schmidt said, shifting in his chair and making it creak. "Do you really think that you can live with someone twenty-four hours a day and they don't know these things. The truth of the matter is that you genuinely love her, and you also have these feelings, and it's okay to have these feelings and it's okay for these feelings to be brought out in the open and dealt with realistically. The fact that you're angry doesn't mean you're going to murder her."

"I just think it would make her feel guilty."

"Then it's her problem not dealing realistically with your feeling. I'm convinced that in your unconscious mind, urinating represents some kind of aggressive action toward Andrea. Feelings and urine held back. I think you would be startled at how much closer you can be when you express your genuine feelings."

"Excuse me," I said. "I have to go urinate."

"That means you have feelings about me or vis-à-vis me that you can't express."

That was undoubtedly true. I sighed, pausing in my trip to the bathroom. "Right now I feel like I have no feelings. I feel subdued. I'm a little sad. And a little jealous that you probably don't have these problems. I feel a little like George Bernard Shaw's feeling about a good bowel movement. I'm beginning to appreciate normal bodily functions."

I thought Schmidt might laugh, or even smile. Instead, he persisted in analysis. "You feel sadness because this is the last session at the end of the summer. And the last overall, because you say you think you are not going to be coming back anymore."

True again. I had seen Schmidt only occasionally, but I thought I had reached, with his help, a point where I understood my relationships well enough to conduct them on my own. I had learned to think about how I talked to our children, to volunteer my feelings before I asked about theirs so that every question wouldn't be an inquisition. I still was learning not to try to contol their choices, but to support the directions they chose. And Andrea and I were closer. Schmidt had helped me see that I sometimes was remote, but her cancer was the galvanizing factor. It had forced me to pay attention, moved me to share the burden of her illness (even though it sometimes made me angry), and emphasized the importance of living in the present.

A more mundane reason I was thinking about dropping my sessions with Schmidt was that Jonathan had decided to end his East Village idyll and return to Columbia. With Joanna starting at Wisconsin, more therapy bills were all I needed.

On the other hand, hearing that I could reveal my anger without feeling guilty, and that I didn't have to choose between my needs and my family's, made me think twice about ending our sessions.

"I haven't made a final decision," I said. "Maybe I'll come back in the fall. In the meantime, I hope you have a good vacation."

I HAD the surgery. The operation was difficult; the surgeon told me afterward in the recovery room that he'd never seen so much blood loss in a prostate procedure.

Recovering, I was in pain for a few days. Andrea was in the hospital, getting her final cycle of chemotherapy. I felt a little let down not to be fussed over by her, but my sister Hinda came up from Princeton and we had lunch together, and Lillian Clyde rescued me for the rest of the week with a copy of *Truman*, which kept me riveted.

Then Andrea was finished with the chemo and getting ready to fly to Wisconsin with Joanna.

"Mommy, you don't have to. I'll be fine. I can handle it. I'll be okay." Joanna's litany of protests fell on deaf ears.

"It's something I want to do, honey. Really, I do," Andrea insisted.

Maybe she was not so ready to let Joanna go into the world as she thought, or as Schmidt wanted her to be.

The reports that came home from their trip were mixed. Joanna described her mother huddled against the side of a building while a stiff wind whipped her clothing and threatened to blow her wig off. Then, once they had moved Joanna's things into her dormitory room, unpacked them and put them away, there was nothing else for Andrea to do. Freshman orientation was full of activities for the incoming students. Joanna wanted to get on with them without worrying about her mother. She wanted to meet her classmates and get to know her new surroundings. She wanted to be free to enter her new world. But she didn't want to hurt Andrea's feelings.

"Mommy, really, you can leave," she finally said. When she told me about it, she said she worried that she was being mean. Andrea took it in stride.

"I had a great time," Andrea said when she got home the next day. "Well, it was a little windy. But when we had Joanna's things put away, she had things to do. I'm proud of her, she's so independent. And so I met Ian and Floriane for dinner. Amani is such a wonderful little boy. He's wary. Well, he would be, wouldn't he? But he likes me, I can tell."

She took her next paycheck to FAO Schwarz and bought Robins's adopted five-year-old a game from which he could assemble pictures from a montage of possibilities.

A month later, she was in remission. I felt good again after a recovery period. Not having to run to the bathroom every half hour made me feel human again.

Normalcy was bursting out all over. Daniel moved to a new job at Sloan-Kettering, out of the Gastroenterology Service into the Genetics Laboratory to do DNA research in solid tumor genetics. I was relieved to have him off my service, not out of any conflict but because I was always uncomfortable that the staff might treat him differently knowing he was my son. He was still living on his own and attending adult curriculum courses at night at NYU in addition to his full-time job.

In October, Andrea and I returned to Madison to attend a parents' weekend with Joanna. We had a good time with her and saw Robins and his family so that Andrea could present her gift to their son.

The next week, we left for Italy.

Chapter

22

W E were filled with anticipation as the 747 waited to take off from Kennedy Airport. Soon the big plane was pushed back from the gate, taxied to the runway, paused, and gathered speed. Only when its wheels lifted off the ground and it banked toward the east did Andrea allow herself the luxury of believing we really had escaped. She leaned back in her seat, closed her eyes, and sighed contentedly. In Italy we would be anonymous, invisible. The cancer couldn't find us there.

We landed in Rome the next morning. Even immigration, customs, and a night of ragged sleep couldn't interfere with the sense that our problems were behind us. We picked up a small rental car and drove south, out of the buzzing traffic of Rome toward Naples. Below Naples, the next dimple in the coastline was the Gulf of Salerno. Positano lay on a peninsula jutting out toward the Isle of Capri. Our guidebook told us the area is called the Amalfi coast, and it must be one of the most beautiful areas on earth. Pastel-colored houses dotted hillsides that plunged down to the blue Mediterranean waters, right out of the picture from the paper.

The staff at Hotel Le Sirenuse greeted us sympathetically after our three-hour drive, and whisked us through a maze of marble hallways to our room. There, a bellhop threw open large French doors to a terrace that looked down the hillside to the sea. The curve of the hillside with its multicolored houses made us feel like spectators in an amphitheater. Capri rose from the sea in the distance beyond the tip of the peninsula.

"Enjoy yourselves, eh?" he told me as he accepted my tip and left us. There was something conspiratorial about his tone and the look he gave me, and I had to think before I remembered what it was. Then I almost laughed out loud.

"What?" Andrea said.

She was wearing a short, dark, curly wig that made her look like an ingenue. "He as much as winked at me. He must have thought you're my mistress. Remember the first time I took you to the opera, and I was self-conscious because you looked so young?"

"So? Let them think what they want," she said, and kissed me.

For the next few days we wandered Positano's steep, narrow streets, browsed in its shops, ate in its small restaurants that were tucked away here and there on the beach and in the hills around the village. Andrea was a picture of youth in shorts, short-sleeved tops, and sneakers. We sat on the terrace, talking and sipping wine, and enjoyed the view propped against the pillows on our king-size bed.

Capri remained on the horizon. We kept saying to each other, "We really should go to Capri." But Positano was simply too enjoyable. One day faded into the next and we were happy to be just where we were, together.

Our togetherness brought to mind our second honeymoon, the winter we were married. Andrea's enthusiasm for the ski trip to Austria masked the fact that she didn't really ski. I spent several days skiing with a group of experts, leaving her with a novice group and an instructor, before I awoke to the fact that she was miserable. Once my eyes were opened, I stopped skiing and spent my time with her. We took chairlifts to sightsee, explored Salzburg and Innsbruck, and had a wonderful time. I had sworn then I would always devote myself to her. But in the intervening years before she got sick, with the ever-increasing responsibilities of children and work, I had reverted to the early days of that ski trip and focused on what I wanted. In Positano, I was reminded once again of the pleasures one finds in partnership, outside oneself.

Andrea spent much of her time drawing. She abandoned her female forms for the subjects at hand — the houses on the hillsides, Capri in the distance, flowers, still lifes of arrangements in our room.

Her eagerness captivated strangers and made her an object of attention among crowds. Her magnetism and appeal transformed her surroundings. One night we entered by chance a small restaurant on the beach. It had warm tile floors and white tablecloths and potted plants and a terrace open to the sea, and we stayed for dinner. She engaged the waiter with her warm smile and friendly eyes. He was her friend within minutes, and for the rest of a long, enchanted evening, accompanied by the sounds of a piano playing softly and the waves on the beach and the feel of soft Mediterranean breezes, he fussed and catered to her through our simple meal of pasta, salad, bread, and wine.

We found simple pleasures at every turn. One day we drove along the Amalfi coast. The road through the mountains was a series of spectacular hairpin turns that first turned away from the sea and then teetered at its edge. Andrea gasped with delight each time the water reappeared below us and we seemed about to leave the road in a steep dive.

The hairpin road took us to Amalfi, where we turned inland. The next town was Ravello. We parked and walked around, seeing what there was to see, and happened into the courtyard of an old building where there was a trattoria. It seemed to be a place the tourists hadn't found. The tables were filled with Italian families and couples. We found a table and time seemed to slow. We lost any sense of having to do anything or go anyplace or see anything. The pleasure of the moment was to sit and eat, to savor tastes and textures, to watch and listen and soak up our surroundings. We left the trattoria two hours later, fresh and relaxed as from a meditation.

The guidebook told us Ravello was known for the ceramics that are made there. We looked at dishes in a little shop. Andrea picked out a pattern of fish and chickens in bright blues and greens and reds, a reflection of her playful nature. She chose dinner and salad and dessert plates, serving platters and even pitchers and arranged to have them shipped home.

"We'll use these when I come home after the transplant," she said. "For a long time, I hope. I'd hate to see you using them with anybody else." She laughed, but I worried there was a morbid undercurrent to her laughter.

We drove to Pompeii another day. Mount Vesuvius rose in the background. The volcano was an apt metaphor for the destruction hanging over Andrea. She hardly seemed to notice. Instead, she insisted that we engage a guide to take us through the ruins of the town that was destroyed in the first century A.D. when Vesuvius erupted. He was a distinguished-looking older man with iron gray hair, and he spoke with his hands, as Andrea did in her dramatic moments. We lost ourselves in the story of Pompeii, and I forgot the metaphor of the volcano.

Positano was a gift. It was something sweet and rare, a series of unsurpassable moments that was our offering to each other. Each step we took, each word we spoke, each heartbeat seemed precious. Leaving chemotherapy, surgery, and all the rest of it behind, even for a week, freed us to pay attention to the moments of consideration, kindness, and love that can raise mere existence to a state of joy.

Then, almost before we knew it, our week in Positano was at an end and we were in the car heading back to Rome. We would have dinner with an old friend of mine and spend the night before catching our return flight the next morning.

Dr. Massimo Crespi and his girlfriend, Claudia Corpetti, picked us up at our hotel. He was the head of the gastrointestinal unit at the Italian National Cancer Institute. We had met over the years at medical meetings and developed a warm relationship. He drove to a trattoria in Rome's Jewish Quarter, next to an old, burned-out synagogue.

The four of us had fun that night. Andrea sparkled amid the restaurant's white stucco walls, the paintings, the candelabra, and flowers on the tables. She organized a picture taken with the waiters. I could tell that Massimo was impressed with her, with the life that bubbled over with every word and gesture, and it made me proud. He told me later that it was her hope that struck him.

We all toasted hope that night. We raised glasses to the optimistic spirit. And that is what Andrea and I carried as we flew home.

N E W York when we returned was everything Positano had not been. It was bustling and intense in the midst of the fall season. Thanksgiving was coming, and Christmas decorations already were up in the department stores. We prepared for Andrea's bone marrow transplant.

The isolation of the transplant would be a sea change from the togetherness we had just enjoyed. The danger of infection dictates a hospital stay of several weeks. Happily, Memorial Sloan-Kettering encourages patients to make their rooms as much like home as possible, and Andrea and I went shopping for small throw rugs, bed coverings, and window treatments.

At a curtain shop on Third Avenue, we discussed curtains, ties, and rods as if we were newlyweds moving into our first apartment.

"What do you think of the beige?" she asked.

"I don't know. I kind of like the fishnet."

"Fishnet's good for stockings, Sid." Andrea gave her husky laugh. "The beige will be brighter. How long should they be? Should the tiebacks match, or contrast? Wait a minute. What kind of cover is going on the bed? We don't want it to clash."

"God forbid it should clash," I said.

At home, I got out the family photo albums and started going through them. Soon I had a selection of photos of Andrea and the two of us together with the children and with friends. Working on the kitchen table, I put them together into bright collages full of memories. We hung these on the walls of her room. We put in a telephone answering machine, so she could screen her calls. As far as I knew, this was a first for hospital rooms.

For a time, all of this time-consuming, harmless busyness distracted us from the dangers ahead. But on the day she entered the hospital, I recalled the words of C. S. Lewis. Lewis, the English Christian theologian who wrote *The Chronicles of Narnia* and many other books and articles, fell in love with an American woman late in his life. When Joy Davidman contracted cancer, Lewis's God was no longer theoretical, but real, and apparently arbitrary. Lewis railed at God for showing him love, then cruelly dashing it. At one phase of her treatment, Lewis wrote that Davidman was "about to be put on the rack again by our wonderful Lord."

I knew his feeling. Andrea faced the pain and nausea of massive chemotherapy, the isolation of her room, the possibility of serious infection. She was about to go on the rack. Yet somehow, she was cheerful and upbeat as she prepared for this new ordeal.

ANDREA received the chemotherapy over five days. A high enough dose of cisplatin to wipe out the bone marrow would have damaged her kidneys, so Fry Casper prescribed carboplatin, the drug Ian Robins had administered with hyperthermia. This she received on the first, third, and fifth days. She received etoposide, or VP-16, at the same times, and on the third and fifth days doses of cyclophosphamide, another anticancer drug, all dripping through the port in her chest while she was under sedation. The dose was four times higher than any she had received before. As it spread through her system, it ravaged healthy and cancer cells alike.

Several days after the blast of the chemo, Andrea's bone marrow was retrieved from its frozen storage and reinfused through her port. To reinfuse it earlier would have allowed the still-potent chemotherapy to kill the stem cells. Now, as the chemo's effects wore off, the healthy marrow would find its way through her bloodstream to her bones, where it would settle in where the blood-producing stem cells normally reside and — we hoped — take hold. As during her earlier chemotherapy regimen, she received daily injections of Neupogen aimed at stimulating the stem cells in the marrow to produce white cells.

We waited. For seven to ten days, until her reinfused marrow started producing the essential blood cells, especially the white cells, she would be a sitting duck for infections.

Visiting Andrea, I had to first wash my hands, then put on a gown, sterile coverings over my shoes, and a mask over my mouth and nose. Jonathan, Daniel, and I, convening for a family visit, looked like workers in a radiation laboratory. Each doctor, nurse, and orderly had to do the same.

Nurses took her blood every day. It was tested for neutrophil cells, the white blood cells that attack invading organisms and are the gauge of her body's ability to fight infections. Andrea waited avidly for each day's neutrophil count, and I posted the results on a chart on the wall. The chart's line rose from zero. Then it was 0.2, then 0.3, then back to 0.2. The goal was 1.0, the watershed mark of 1,000 neutrophils per cubic centimeter. At this point, the threat of infection would be largely over.

All the horrors of chemotherapy, the hair falling out, the nausea, are paradise next to what can happen to a body unable to ward off infections. The unresistant body can be infected by itself. The skin, the mouth, the vagina, the stool, all carry bacteria and fungi by the trillions that have the potential to infect the body. Normally, these organisms are contained in the areas where they originate. If they try to invade the tissues and cross into the bloodstream they are attacked and killed by the infection-fighting white cells.

In the white cells' absence, the bacteria and fungi enter the tissues unchecked and spread quickly through the bloodstream. They can attack all the organs of the body, producing mouth sores, abscesses, kidney infections, infections of the heart valve, brain abscesses.

Andrea's fever came without warning on the seventh day. She weakened rapidly, and soon could not sit up in bed. The staff, which had been vigilant, began watching her signs with grim intensity. The fever worsened, and there was no time to seek out its cause. She had to be bombarded with antibiotics that attacked every possibility.

Amphotericin B, an antifungal medicine, was part of the mix. Gallows humor in the medical profession has dubbed this powerful drug the "shake and bake" medicine because of its horrendous side effects. Patients suffer high fevers and shake uncontrollably. They say the cure is almost worse than the disease.

Andrea was hit with huge doses of this antibiotic cocktail. The aftermath was more frightening than her swollen, comalike state after the hyperthermia, more frightening than her blistering fever after the interferon. She tossed in the bed, her teeth chattering, her arms and legs jerking, and her hands fluttering with a mad palsy. Her head thrashed from side to side. I tried to give her water, but her head jerked away from the cup I held to her cracked lips.

It was hard to watch. I knew it must have been harder to endure. She truly had been placed on the rack.

The nurses were angels. They were incredible, as they had been during each of her hospitalizations, but now they contended with a spider's web of tubes descending from an IV pole from which hung six or seven bags of fluids — antibiotics, blood plasma, blood platelets, saline, nutrition. Each tube ran to the main line that fed into her port through an automatic pump set at a certain delivery speed. Everything had to be timed exactly; some medicines could not be mixed with others, and each dose had to be checked. Fry Casper and Andrea's other doctors checked her condition several times a day, but a nurse was always there. The nurse-to-patient ratio after an involved and risky procedure like a bone marrow transplant is one nurse to two patients. In Andrea's case, I thought they were the keys to her survival. They certainly were the key to mine, acting as my ad hoc psychotherapists during the times she was at her worst.

Several times over three days, she was hit with the "shake and bake" treatment. She thrashed in torture each time until, on the third day, her palsied hand jerking in mine and the fever descending over her, she cried, "Stop it, just stop it. Sid, make them stop. I can't take it anymore. Please, I'd rather die."

The nurse told her she had just received the final treatment.

Analysis showed that her bloodstream had been infected by candida, or monilia, the same fungus that causes vaginitis in women. This irritating but usually minor fungus infection, entering a bloodstream without the white cells to fight back, had almost been a killer.

Once the infection had been stemmed, Andrea recovered quickly. Her neutrophil count that tracked her white cells rose; the lines I drew on the chart on her wall climbed steadily higher, to 0.7, then 0.8. Then I drew the line that crossed the 1.0 threshold, and we breathed more easily at last.

Chapter

23

I PRAYED during this time. Sitting in Andrea's room while she shuddered from the antibiotics, I prayed for her and asked God to let me concentrate on her and pour my energy and attention into helping her recover from her transplant and its horrible aftermath. She was the most important thing right now, and I prayed that there would be no distractions.

She was still in the worst throes of her infection when I received a call from her sister, Marsha, one morning in my office. She and I also had drawn closer since Andrea's illness.

"Sid, how is she doing?" Marsha asked.

I told her about the infection, and the cure that seemed even worse.

"Then don't tell her this until the time is right, but our father died."

"What happened?" I asked.

"He just wore out. He was eighty-eight, you know. He'd been going downhill ever since Mom died."

I had had some vague inkling, and Andrea had, too. Without Helen, Michael Bloom had withered in the last fifteen months. For much of that time, he'd been living with Marsha and her husband in New Jersey.

Each time I thought angrily of his failure to back Andrea, when she was a child, against her mother, I thought also of his grief. It was like the grief I feared, and sympathy replaced my anger.

I agonized over whether to tell Andrea. Eventually, I decided to wait until she was in better shape.

Daniel and I planned to attend the funeral. Jonathan also wanted to come, but I discouraged him.

"Why not?" he said.

"You're in the middle of midterms. You really don't need to deal with this right now. Don't worry about it. Daniel and I will go."

My prayer for stability had turned me back into the controlling father, the man who had to manage everything and who apologized when the weather was out of his control. Daniel and I attended the funeral by ourselves. In my wish to protect Jonathan from the trauma of his grandfather's funeral and maintain some stability around him, I deprived him of something more valuable — a sharing of the family's sadness. Jonathan was angry, and I realized later my mistake.

When I later told Andrea, she nodded and mused, "I guess I expected it. Poor Dad, he didn't have anything to live for without her." She harbored none of the anger toward him that she had for her mother.

AT the end of three weeks, I took down the curtains and collages and unplugged the answering machine, and took Andrea home. She pushed herself to get well enough to attend the Thanksgiving dinner we shared each year with our friends of more than twenty years, Sandy and Maurice Steinberg. Andrea and Sandy were the basis of the friendship. They had met soon after the Steinbergs moved into our apartment building, when Sandy had a one-year-old and Daniel had just been born. They were sitting on a wall outside the building with the boys, and Sandy said, "What's his name?"

"Daniel. And yours?"

"He's Daniel, too."

They had been pregnant with their second sons together, and Jonathan and Michael Steinberg were almost the same age. Andrea and Sandy had watched each other's children when they were young, and in a real way, our families had grown up together. Now they lived in Great Neck. We were accustomed to Thanksgiving at their house, and in the summer they usually came to a Fourth of July celebration at our Amagansett beach house.

"I don't see how you'll possibly be well enough," Fry Casper said. "It's not unusual for patients to take months before they're up to speed again."

But Andrea was determined, and defiant. Fry had told her to stay away from her beloved Daisy, pointing out that she still was vulnerable to infection and that handling animals increased the risk.

"Daisy's as clean as a person," Andrea said, cuddling the tiny dog.

I could only believe that the comfort of animal companions had therapeutic value, too.

We traditionally exchanged gifts with the Steinbergs on Thanksgiving. Andrea went shopping on Wednesday before the holiday. She came home with an armful of shopping bags. By the time she had picked out the outfit she wanted to wear, I could see she was exhausted.

We closed our eyes and meditated together for half an hour. When she still looked drained, I said, "Look, let's not go tomorrow. There's no sense pushing yourself. Sandy and Maurice will understand."

Andrea glared at me, her eyes under hairless eyebrows accusing me of losing faith in her. "We're going. We'll have a good time, too. You'll see." I saw in her, as I had before we left for Italy, that determination to reach a goal that kept some patients going.

She rose on Thanksgiving morning and summoned some hidden reserve of energy. Her mood grew lighter as we headed out to the island with Daniel and Jonathan, and Joanna, who had flown in from Madison the night before. At the door, Sandy gathered Andrea into a hug and said, "We didn't think you'd make it."

"They pumped me full of the most unbelievable stuff," Andrea said. "But I told Sid, good friends are the best medicine."

As we sat down to the feast before us, I said a traditional Jewish blessing that deepened the meaning of the holiday:

"Blessed art thou, O lord our God, king of the universe, who has kept us in life, sustained us, and enabled us to reach this day."

This brief, heartfelt blessing was one of my favorites, and weeper that I am, saying it brought tears to my eyes. There was so much in my heart. The last months had tested us, but they also had made us mindful of our blessings, not least the dawn of each new day. Our children were around us, they were healthy, we were alive and all together. Our gifts were abundant.

After dinner, the kids retired to watch football and the parents stayed around the table. Andrea drove the conversation. She was a dynamo. I watched her with pride and concealed amazement, as she drew from our friends details of their lives, displayed her interest in them and their activities, never dwelling on the cancer or the torture she had recently been through. My love for her surged.

I loved her because she was my Andrea. Unlike her parents and her friends, I had never given her a nickname. Not Andi or Annie, which her parents called her, or Cookie, used by Marsha and some of her friends. Nicknames can be terms of affection, but I had always loved the sound of Andrea too much to diminish it in any way. She was my life, my love, my wife, and I loved her for her courage, determination, and willpower, and the energy she transmitted to everybody in the room. Her vitality spilled over and sparked our gathering; there was enough for everyone. I had seen glimmers of this energy before — our honeymoon in Nassau, and the charged night at the roulette table, with the people touching her for luck — but never so much of it as now. I saw her as a life force, capable of transforming herself as well as those around her. I wondered if she knew how much her quest for healing had also transformed me.

Change had come across a wide spectrum of my life. That her cancer had brought it was not true in every case. I would have deciphered fatherhood without it, for example, helped by my talks with Dr. Schmidt. But Andrea's cancer, and her response to it, had awakened me to new possibilities as a husband and a doctor. I paid more attention now. I was more alert to the possibilities of our relationship. I saw that time was too precious to plan special events for the distant future. Special moments were waiting every day. I thought I listened better and was a better, more responsive husband. She, as a patient who took control of her options, had shown me how I, as a doctor, might improve other patients' chances by bringing them and their spouses fully into a treatment plan. And she had shown me, in her explorations of meditation and in the Bible reading and prayer we did together, the complements to conventional medicine that could do so much to improve a patient's prospects and quality of life. I was open to new possibilities in medicine, and even if I was unconvinced of the value of interferon or vitamin supplements, I saw that, in many cases, what gave a patient hope was what a doctor should encourage.

These gifts, too, I added to my list of blessings.

Thanksgiving, and then Hanukkah, Christmas, and Pat Kadvan's New Year's Eve party welcoming 1993. It was the second New Year we had welcomed since Andrea's initial death sentence. Andrea's LDH levels and CT scans continued to look good. Her hair returned, in childlike down at first, then dark and thick as it had been before the chemotherapy, but with a white streak in the front that people said made her look like Loretta Young. From the six months I first thought she had to live, she had survived two years.

Chapter

24

WITH Andrea once again in remission, Dr. Schmidt wanted her to try another immunostimulant to replace the interferon and somatostatin.

"You still need all the weapons you can get," he told us one day that winter. I hadn't returned to Schmidt on my own, but continued, now and then, to go with Andrea. "Why don't you check out DHEA?"

I always bridled at Schmidt's suggestions, but I tried to be open-minded. In any case Andrea, once Schmidt had mentioned a new drug, invariably wanted to know more. DHEA is ubiquitous at health food and vitamin stores today, but early in 1993 I had to return to Sloan-Kettering's medical library, the computer, and the phones to research this new suggestion. What I found surprised me. Schmidt again was up-to-date on the latest medical research. A flurry of new studies suggested that DHEA, a steroid hormone whose function had been little known until recently, might in fact be a medical treasure trove.

DHEA, or dehydroepiandrosterone, is similar to estrogen, testosterone, and progesterone, but with its own biological effect. It is produced and secreted by the adrenal glands, in greater quantities than any other hormone they produce. Researchers had been uncovering links between DHEA and the prevention and treatment of a wide range of disorders, including heart disease, high cholesterol, diabetes, obesity, cancer, Alzheimer's disease, memory disturbances, and immune system disorders, including AIDS and chronic fatigue. Studies hinted that it might also increase the body's immune responsiveness against viral and bacterial infections. It was seen as a potential antiaging hormone and as a means of preventing osteoporosis, the bone loss suffered by older women as the result of calcium deficiencies that come when their estrogen levels decline after menopause.

Animal studies with DHEA had shown anticancer activity. Mice given cancer-causing chemicals, then treated with DHEA, had shown a delayed onset of their cancers. DHEA also had inhibited the development of liver cancer in rats treated with chemical carcinogens.

Research into DHEA was just beginning to unfold, and some data was ambiguous. Limited studies with patients suggested that DHEA might have been a factor in the prevention of breast cancer, while other researchers argued that supplemental DHEA, by increasing hormonal metabolism, could actually increase the risk of hormone-dependent cancers like breast cancer in women and prostate cancer in men. The hormone's role and potential benefits in cancer prevention and treatment were so far only tempting possibilities, while its downside was equally uncertain. Much work remained to be done.

Schmidt, however, urged Andrea to use anything that had potential. He used the by-now-familiar military metaphor: "Add it to your armory. You need every weapon and every bit of ammunition in this war."

Andrea agreed. She concluded that the possibilities outweighed the risks.

The problem then was, where to get it.

THERE was no such thing as a DHEA prescription. It had not yet shown up on the shelves of health food stores. Synthetic DHEA was available in only a handful of pharmacies in the United States. It wasn't illegal, but it had not been approved for sale by the Food and Drug Administration, and you had to know a pharmacist who stocked it in compound form or someone at a clinical laboratory who could acquire it from a pharmaceutical manufacturer as a reagent for chemical assays.

Schmidt knew a pharmacy in Greenwich Village that had a large AIDS clientele. That he had such a resource had long ago ceased to be surprising, but I still marveled at the extent of his network. He knew not only the AIDS treatments and medications that had a potential against cancer, but where they could be found. At the pharmacy, we learned that we could get DHEA in powder form. We would have to make up our own capsules. Andrea would take two a day, one in the morning and one at night.

The pharmacist arrived at our apartment one evening about seven. He was a pleasant, soft-spoken man, casually dressed, someone you wouldn't notice in a crowd. He had brought his girlfriend; they were on their way to dinner.

"Here we are," he said, pulling a large jar of powdered DHEA out of a plastic shopping bag. With it, he had a supply of empty gelatin capsules. "Let me see." He looked around. "I wanted to show you how to get it in the capsules."

I led the way into the den. The girlfriend immediately admired Andrea's drawings, and the two of them started talking while he shook out some of the white powder onto the glass desktop. Using a small pharmacist's spatula, he filled half of a capsule with the powder, then capped it with the other half. It all took a matter of seconds.

"There," he said. "Now you try it."

He had done it with the deftness of a magician making a coin disappear, and I wanted to watch him again. After he filled two more, I gave it a try. I managed to scatter powder all over the desktop and mangle several capsules. I might as well have been wearing mittens on my hands.

He looked at his girlfriend. She shrugged. Andrea laughed her wicked laugh. "He's not an eye surgeon, he's a gastroenterologist," she said.

After I muffed several more attempts, the pharmacist gently took my place. He sat at the desk and filled capsules while I stood in the door and watched. His hands moved with an unconscious grace. The analogy was not a production line robot, but a craftsman at one with his work. He filled capsule after capsule without apparent effort, talking all the while about his father. "I loved him," he said. "He saw most of this century. He always used to talk about the things he'd seen. All the wonderful, crazy things. He died of cancer. This might have helped him, I don't know." Andrea and the girlfriend talked, too, but I was too fascinated with the pharmacist to hear what they were saying. His hands moved like little dancing puppets moved by unseen strings. I was mesmerized. I forgot my fear of yet another drug, another step outside Andrea's protocol.

Time passed. The hour grew late. The powder in the jar diminished while the pile of capsules grew. Now and then he dumped them into a smaller glass jar I had brought from the kitchen. When he had made several hundred, he stopped, poured the remaining powder back into the jar and gathered up the empty capsules. I reached for my checkbook.

"How much do I owe you?" I asked. If the cost of interferon was any guide, it would be a lot.

He smiled. "Not a thing."

"What do you mean? You brought all this stuff, you did all this work, you spent all this time."

He shrugged. "I'm happy to do it. I hope it works out for the two of you. We've just got to do these things for each other."

We saw them to the door. He shook my hand and hugged Andrea and the girlfriend gave us both hugs. "Take care of yourself," he said to Andrea. "You can beat this thing. I know lots of people who have done it."

The door closed and Andrea and I turned to each other with tears in our eyes. "There are such good people in the world," she said.

"I know," I said. "Sometimes you forget they're out there." But such people seemed to be the rule in the realms of medicine Andrea and I had been exploring. I thought how much conventional medicine could relearn about showing sympathy, generosity, and care.

DANIEL moved in March to a new apartment at Thirtieth and Third, in Murray Hill. Since he was no longer working on the gastroenterology service, and Andrea was at the hospital only for her monthly CT scans and to have blood drawn for testing, neither of us saw him as often. When he invited us to see his new place, Andrea bought a plant as a housewarming present and we drove downtown.

We were greeted at the door by a moist billow of aromas.

"What's that?" Andrea stepped past Daniel and gathered the aromas toward her with both hands. "It smells like a forest. You're not growing marijuana, are you, Daniel?"

Daniel laughed and led us along scent trails of moss and cedar and tree bark to the kitchen. Steam rose from a pot boiling on the stove. The bubbling mixture was visceral and dark. "It's Chinese herbs," he said.

"What are they for?"

"Originally to make my collarbone heal faster. These are to prevent the flu."

Daniel had told us of his lessons in Wing Chun, a Chinese martial art also called short-armed boxing. Andrea and I were fascinated, because there was a meditation component in his Wing Chun practice. He had observed our increasingly deeper explorations into meditation and took pains to explain the principles of Chi Gong meditation. As he related it, Chi Gong adherents believe the body is an empty chamber of energy, in which balance must be achieved. He showed us Chi Gong meditations in a variety of standing and sitting positions that were about learning to balance and feel your energy.

Earlier, Daniel had broken his collarbone when he rode his bicycle into a New York City pothole, and the only person who could set it was his Wing Chun master. Three conventional doctors — "Western medicine doctors," as he put it, or doctors like myself — had failed. The master then sent him to an herbal shop in Chinatown for a prescription that would help the break mend quickly.

He rolled his shoulders and moved his arms with no apparent pain. "Herbs," he said. "You should try them. Chinese herbal medicine is as effective as anything you can find in Western medicine."

Andrea listened raptly as Daniel described the potential and variety of herbal medicine, and the rapid healing of his shoulder. All I knew about herbal medicine was that it had a long history of use in Asia and a growing number of Western devotees.

A week later, buttoned up against a raw March wind, we followed Daniel down Elizabeth Street in Chinatown toward a shop with the single English word, "Herbs," under Chinese characters on its marquee.

Inside the small shop, glass shelves overflowed with packaged remedies and a long counter set off a working area and tiers of square wooden drawers. Men and women in white coats — I didn't know whether to call them herbalists or druggists — moved busily behind the counter, taking herbs from the drawers and combining them on plastic placemats on the countertop. An old-fashioned mortar and pestle was set into one end of the counter. The workers measured the proportions of the herbs by eye or using hand-held brass scales.

Daniel said we wanted to talk with someone about a prescription. After a short wait, a small man in a white coat appeared and introduced himself. "Hello, I'm Dr. Chen." He gave a slight bow.

I shook his hand. "I'm Dr. Winawer. This is my wife, Andrea. She has cancer. Our son tells us you may have something that can help."

Dr. Chen studied us, deciding if we were sincere. Then he nodded and led the way to a tiny examination room behind the main room of the shop. It contained a narrow cot, covered with a white sheet, set against the wall under a chart of acupuncture points on a naked Chinese man. Overhead, sagging plywood shelves held plastic bags bulging with dried herbs. A crooked piece of wire strayed above the cot from head to foot, holding a makeshift curtain that could be pulled for privacy. In the wall abutting the main room of the shop, a small fan-shaped window showed the backs of shelves and more packaged remedies.

The herbal doctor offered Andrea a chair, then sat down himself on a chair wedged between a small cabinet and the cot. I stood in the doorway. There was no room to close the door. I wondered what we were doing there. What did this have to do with the medicine I knew?

Dr. Chen's manner, however, put me at ease. He had a healing aura or, as Daniel put it, "a good oneness with the universe" that came from being calm, deliberate, and quietly self-assured. He took a pen from the pocket of the white shirt he wore, open at the collar, under his white coat and prepared to take notes on lined paper in a spiral notepad.

The doctor asked Andrea about her medical history. He wrote in Chinese characters as she described her cancer, her treatments, and the bone marrow transplant. Now and then he nodded. Then he asked me to come into the room and close the door. I squeezed in, and he instructed Andrea to lie down on the cot for an examination. She raised her blouse, and he pressed his hand against her abdomen over her liver.

"No heat. Not big," he said. "You say there was a biopsy?"

"I'm afraid so," Andrea said.

Dr. Chen expressed surprise. "No cancer now."

"No," Andrea said. "I'm in remission. I'd like to stay that way."

"I understand," Dr. Chen said quietly. As Andrea tucked in her blouse, he turned to a clean page in his notepad and wrote several lines of characters, then tore it out and handed it to her. "This is for your immunity. Boil for half an hour and drink two cups a day, but take your other medications, too."

We handed the prescription to one of the herbalists in the front of the store. She took herbs from several drawers, mixed them on the counter, and shook them into small brown paper bags. A two-week supply, and a porcelain pot to boil them in, cost about $100.

"But what's in it?" I asked.

Frank Lin, the shop's manager, came forward to translate the Chinese. "This is a common prescription for stimulating the immune system. Codonopsis, astragalus, and dan kwei, they're all roots, and lin zi, which is a fungus."

"What else does Dr. Chen prescribe for cancer?"

Lin described a combination of herbs, roots, and fungi that would help the body balance itself to prevent cancer, another that would flush the intestines to ward off colon cancer, another that would adjust the metabolism. Other herbal prescriptions, he said, would offset the effects of chemotherapy, stimulate the appetite, help digestion, and counteract nausea.

Andrea put water on to boil as soon as we got home. Soon our apartment, too, was smelling like a forest. The viscous soup created from boiling the herb mixture wasn't particularly appealing. Andrea made a face when she drank each cup, but she drank it faithfully. She was a therapeutic nihilist when it came to drugs like pain relievers and antihistamines, but the herbs were natural, and therefore, okay.

"Make no mistake, those herbs are drugs," Ian Robins exploded when Andrea told him she was using herbal therapy to stimulate her immune system. "I'm glad you weren't taking them when you were in my program."

My own view was less critical. I was amused to think that Ian, whose "radical" hyperthermia program had caused me such misgivings two years earlier, had turned out to be a more conventional doctor than the one I was becoming. I was no expert on herbs just because Andrea used them. My understanding, and Western medicine's in general, of herbs and their healing powers remained relatively unsophisticated. Nevertheless, it was clear, from herbal medicine's long history of use and growing popularity, and the growing use of natural remedies, that nature contains vast potential for treatments and cures both known and unknown. Digitalis is the most obvious example. This commonly prescribed medication for heart diseases is made from the dried leaf of the common foxglove.

Later, I would find myself prescribing Saint-John's-wort for an elderly patient whose problems with acid reflux would not respond to conventional medicine because of his underlying depression, for which he refused to seek therapy. The herb, from a flowering green plant, is like Prozac without the side effects.

Ultimately, Andrea stopped brewing and drinking the herbal soup prescribed by Dr. Chen. She continued to drink green herbal tea she bought at the Chinatown shop, but she didn't have a strong conviction that the herbal soup was helping her, and she already was taking an immunostimulant with DHEA. That, and the fact that it depressed her appetite when she had always struggled to take in enough calories, made her give it up.

Nevertheless, Eastern medicine's centuries of extensive and knowledgeable use of herbs bears further exploration by Western medicine.

Chapter

25

ANDREA continued to see Dr. Schmidt three times a week. I had powerfully opposing feelings about this. I saw the great improvement evidenced by her taking control of her treatment options and the power that was manifest in the lifestyle changes she had made. However, nearly ten years now into psychotherapy — and more than two years after she felt that she had been ready to phase it out before the cancer intervened — she still was struggling through her inner conflicts. It had gone on endlessly, without resolution. I understood her need and supported her in all she did. At the same time, I would have liked to see an end to it.

But Andrea was locked in her relationship with Schmidt. It was an endless cycle in which she needed his reassurance to define her. She went to him to get her psychological gas tank filled. He reinforced her belief in the power of the mind. He gave her the midcourse corrections she needed, helped her work through issues that stood in her way, and she often came home pumped up and believing again. The level of hope these sessions gave her stood against the bleak portrait of the so-called cancer personality.

Her hope was great, but so was the burden of her expectations.

"The most important news is that I've been working on my imaging," she announced to Schmidt at the beginning of a session in April, one of those she kept on tape. "I've been seeing a lot of little men with mops and brooms, in my liver, and they're cleaning and washing my liver.

"And my LDH, I'm imaging one-forty-eight," she continued. "That's pretty good, one-forty-eight. I've decided the next time, it's going to be one-forty-five. One-forty-five, that sounds good, doesn't it? Do you think it will work?" There was that smoky laughter in her voice, but also the need to hear him say yes.

"It's called mop therapy," he said, and they both laughed. Humor had been a rare commodity in my relationship with Schmidt, and as far as I knew, in Andrea's as well. This was something new.

They talked more about her cancer. He seemed surprised she still had the port and questioned the need for it, since she was in remission and no longer taking chemo. She told him her white cell count was 4.3.

Her infection-fighting white cells had slowly increased after the purposeful destruction and replacement of her bone marrow. Four-point-three, or 4,300 white cells per cubic centimeter, was well above the 1,000 cell threshold at which she was out of danger from opportunistic infections after the transplant. But it was still, in Schmidt's view, too low. His chair creaked and pages riffled as he apparently checked a medical reference. "Normal is four to eleven," he said. "You're just squeaking by."

More unexpected, but no longer surprising, expertise from Schmidt.

WHAT came next prompted me to believe that Andrea was beginning, after all, to resolve her conflicted feelings about the children's independence. She had been furious that Daniel had chosen to attend a Passover seder at my sister Joyce's on Long Island, rather than with us at her sister Marsha's in New Jersey. It was an innocent choice; Daniel loved the give-and-take he always had with Joyce and her four kids. Nevertheless, Andrea had expressed her anger to Schmidt.

"You were the queen of hostility," the psychiatrist told her. His tone was gentler than on the other tapes. It went with the humor. I wondered if he was being easier on Andrea because she was getting it, at last. Or maybe something was happening in his own life that was causing him to mellow. "You were saying, 'Off with his head. Off with his intelligence,'" he continued. "But he's an independent creature. He's supposed to decide which seder he wants to attend, and you have to accept that."

Andrea agreed. "He just has to go ahead and take care of his life. He has to take care of himself and decide what he wants to do. I've been working on that. And it turned out that we had a wonderful seder without him."

She turned to discussing Jonathan, whom she had pushed into early achievements such as math lessons at two and a half, violin lessons, and computer courses in the sixth grade. "I just pushed him into everything, because he could do those things. But I stopped. I have let go of a lot of that. He stopped going to Columbia, and I got over that. Living down in the East Village, I was okay with that. Every time I wanted to push him, I said to myself, 'You know what, if you want to take a course at Columbia, go take a course at Columbia. If you want to learn the computer, go learn the computer.' I took it out of him and put it into myself. I've given up my dreams of what I hoped he would be."

"They're called displacements," said Dr. Schmidt. "The ambitions you had to succeed, you placed on him."

"It doesn't work," Andrea said. "I see it, and I've given it up. But now, he won't let me close to him. He's afraid it will compromise his independence. He doesn't call, and when I talk to him, I can't even ask him how he is, or where he goes, or what he does."

"He's not rejecting you. He's rejecting your intrusiveness," Schmidt said. "It's easy. All you have to do is do nothing. That's what he wants."

Andrea wanted to get it right, but it was hard to let go. "At times, I become afraid that I'll never see him again."

"You are not entitled to have your kids around forever. Your only agreement was to bring them up the best you can and that's it."

"But not seeing him feels like a failure on my part."

"Why do you think having your kids hanging around forever is a sign of success? It's a sign of dismal failure."

"It's not what I expected."

"You expected Mommy and Brainy Child to be blissfully together forever."

"Yes."

"No, it ain't so. This is reality."

"But it would be nice."

"Only if it's what you both want."

"I thought the success of raising a child would mean that he would want to be with you."

"Why do you think in terms of success and failure? Success and failure only counts in sports, where there are winners and losers. Relationships are grayer."

Yes, I thought. How many people find the perfect love that they expect? How many dreams come true in just the way that they're imagined? Success brings disappointment because it is not all that we anticipate. If only we could recognize the success in the unexpected, find the pearl in the moment, then we might find fulfillment. Suddenly, I felt a blinding stab of love for Andrea that gave way to revelation. What matters is only that you care, and that you try. We both cared, we both were trying, and I loved her so desperately in that moment that nothing else mattered. We both wanted to get it right, with each other and the children, and that we stumbled, that we took two steps forward and one back, well, that just placed us with the vast legions of humanity. We were imperfect people trying to be less imperfect, and we were doing it together. I loved her so much I cried.

The tape continued. Dr. Schmidt, continuing his gentle tone, referred back to Andrea's image of little men scrubbing her liver. "One day," he said, "you'll be able to image your independent child."

As she was leaving, Schmidt asked her if she had enough DHEA capsules. "The pharmacist has been away. He's coming back, but if you need them, I can let you have some of mine."

"No thanks, I've got plenty," she said. "I didn't know you were taking DHEA."

Chapter

26

ANDREA'S CT scans and blood tests continued to show no sign of cancer. She felt vulnerable, however. The bone marrow transplant really had been her last chance at a cure. Platinum-based chemotherapy, after miraculously working a second time, would not work again, with or without hyperthermia. She continued to take DHEA, vitamin supplements, and at the time was still taking her herbal prescription. She power walked, read the Bible, meditated, held in her mind's eye the image of her liver being scrubbed clean, and went for supportive therapy to Schmidt. There was nothing else for her to do.

We tried not to watch the calendar. But it was impossible not to look ahead to a time when we might believe the cancer was gone and she was cured.

"I'm in my ninth month of remission," she said in early May. "I'm thinking of October-November as a kind of a pivotal time. I feel I have to get through to October or November. It will be a year since my transplant. Do you think I'll be cured, if there's no cancer then?"

I thought ahead. With cancer, you never know. "A year will be an excellent milestone," I said.

But Positano reminded us not to wait. We needed to live, to experience moments and create memories, not wait to learn what the future would bring. We both had always wanted to explore the south of France, but kept putting it off. In May, we waited no longer.

We flew into Nice, arriving on a bright Mediterranean morning with ten days ahead of us with no set plans and nothing to do except drive from village to village. We picked up a rental car. Signs beckoned us to Monaco, Cannes, and Saint-Tropez, but hectic vacations and obligatory sightseeing were things of the past. We drove west to Aix-en-Provence. There, we stopped to stroll its wide, tree-lined boulevard, the Cours Mirabeau, and ate a long lunch in crisp spring sunshine while we surveyed the passing scene. From there, we drove on to Arles.

When we reached our hotel, I opened the trunk and stood for a moment, transfixed with disappointment. The small overnight bags with our vouchers, passports, and toiletries were missing. Apparently I had left the trunk unlocked, and a thief had done his work while we were enjoying our leisurely lunch.

"Oh, Sid, what are we going to do?" Andrea said, momentarily distraught as we surveyed the damage.

"I don't know," I said, "but we'll figure it out."

She closed her eyes and took a deep breath right there in the parking lot. After a minute she opened her eyes and said, "Wait a minute. You know, I really hated that passport photograph. This is not such a bad thing. Look at it this way, we're in France. If a woman has to lose her makeup, France is the place, right?"

I laughed in spite of myself.

In times past, given my tendency to worry, this might have been a serious challenge. On our healing path, she was right, it was an opportunity. A call home from the hotel desk to our travel agent replaced our vouchers via the hotel fax machine. The stolen passports required a detour to Marseilles and the U.S. Consulate the next day. This gave us a chance to explore the crowded, storied port city in search of bouillabaisse. We struck the mother lode in a small cafe overlooking the harbor. Andrea, as usual, captivated the waiter, who passionately recited the virtues of our sumptuous meal. In the afternoon, our passports replaced, Andrea's minimal makeup replenished, and the car's trunk safely locked, we went on our way.

The Provençal countryside amazed us with its beauty. We kept to small winding roads between the towns and small villages, past fields of flowers and picturesque old houses perched on hillsides. We saw the light that drew the Impressionists to Arles and the surrounding area. Colors shifted and deepened as the sun moved across the sky: meadows showed new greens, yellows, oranges, and golds; fields of flowers splashed hotter pinks and reds; green trees hung against a backdrop of blue sky streaked with white clouds; plowed earth oozed rich blacks and browns.

Andrea, who normally left the photos to me, took the camera and called out for me to stop the car at each new vista. She also kept her drawing materials handy and sketched in pencil the profiles of the folding hills.

We knew the towns and hotels where we would be each night. Between them, our itinerary shifted moment to moment. We turned onto roads that just looked promising and followed them. We stopped at restaurants with dogs in the yard, lingered over meals, browsed in shops that caught our eye. Ranging west into the Languedoc and the walled medieval city of Carcassonne, we found an exquisite restaurant where we whiled away an afternoon just sipping wine and talking.

The tables slowly emptied until we were alone in the restaurant. The waiter and the rest of the staff seemed in no hurry to have us leave. Soon, two small children ran into the restaurant followed by a woman. A smile broke onto the waiter's face and he embraced his children and his wife. The younger of the children, a girl, looked around the room and spotted us. She kept looking back, staring at Andrea until it became obvious and her mother spoke to her. But she couldn't stop, and Andrea suddenly figured it out.

"It's the streak in my hair," she said.

She caught the girl's eye when she looked again, and beckoned her. "Come on. You can look, it's okay."

The family talked, then the waiter came holding his shy daughter's hand. The girl took timid steps, but her fascination drew her forward. When they reached us, Andrea leaned forward and took the girl's hands. "Do you like my hair?" she said.

One small hand withdrew from Andrea's and reached up to touch the silver streak of hair. Andrea lowered her head and the girl combed the streak with her fingers. Suddenly she laughed with delight and cried, "*Oui. C'est epatant!*" She clasped Andrea's face in both hands, kissed her, and gave her a hug. Then she ran giggling back to her mother.

"She said it is wonderful," the waiter said gravely.

"Oh, my," said Andrea. "Oh, my," and looked in her purse for a tissue. "Tell her she is wonderful, too."

We settled our bill and the waiter left with his family. Andrea and the girl waved goodbye to each other, solemnly, knowing they would never see each other again. We sat for another moment quietly. When we finally emerged onto the ancient street, it felt as if we had left some stirring opera or a worship service, or had awakened from a dream.

"That," Andrea said, "that was a gift."

Nothing duplicated the wonder of that moment, but we had many pleasures. We felt in no hurry to do anything, to follow any set requirements. Not feeling that we had to rush from cathedral to castle to museum, we were able to pay attention to the commonplace. The result was that quality of mindfulness — an awareness of natural beauty that surrounded us, the personal warmth of the people we encountered, the food we ate and the wine we drank — that made each day surrender its meaning in a cascade of sparkling gems. Feeling free to move with our instincts, we decided in Avignon that we didn't like the hotel we had booked and moved on the spur of the moment to another. The Hotel d'Europe, with Aubusson tapestries and antiques and works of art and lots of character, better satisfied our mood.

Andrea smiled the whole time. I never saw her without a smile on her face. She was buoyant. Like a small child chasing butterflies, she was taken by whatever interested her, and I saw over and over how attention to the moments enhanced our hours and our days. We held hands a lot, like honeymooners.

But my legacy of worrying gave me no peace. One day, I was admiring her hair, with its striking white streak, thinking of the little girl, and felt a sudden chill as I wondered if everything else in her body also was growing again. Were the cancer cells growing along with her hair?

I kept my worries to myself.

"see what I'm calling it?" Andrea held up the album she made of our photos from Provence. She had written, "The best trip of our lives," inside the cover.

We were home and full of hope. Summer was approaching. Joanna soon would be home from Wisconsin. Hope vied with the reality that Andrea was still in danger. If only we could get through to the fall. Looking ahead, we also had to remember to look to the things that were important in our lives — children, friends, each other. Hope for the future and the possibility of remission or cure enabled us to enjoy life fully in the present. One moment would lead to the next, and the next.

The summer began. We resumed our weekends at Amagansett, long days cooled by ocean breezes, evenings together, visits from the kids, long walks by the sea, Daisy scampering after birds, Andrea carrying the tiny dog when she was exhausted.

July Fourth approached. We got ready for Sandy and Maurice Steinberg's visit, our annual reciprocation for the Thanksgivings we traditionally spent with them. Andrea put special care into the planning. She shopped for several meals and bought a red-white-and-blue tablecloth, American flag napkins and plates, and a flag to hang from the deck. Before we left the city, she stopped by Bob Kurtz's office to have blood drawn for another LDH test.

"I'm not going to worry about it," she said as we drove east, Jonathan and Joanna with us in the car and Daniel planning to come out by train in the morning. "I'm just going to have a good time."

The Steinbergs arrived with their sons on Saturday and until they left on Sunday night we had an old-fashioned Fourth of July, barbecuing on the deck, watching the fireworks that spouted like colored fountains over the South Fork, and talking long into the night. The weekend was especially warm in terms of the shared friendship. Memories of holiday weekends past flowed like good wine. No matter what personal turmoil we were going through, we all had reasons to be grateful, and we toasted many Independence Days to come.

Sunday was the fourth, Monday the day stores and offices were closed, so when the phone rang on Monday morning I answered it, expecting to hear Sandy or Maurice thanking us for the weekend. I heard Bob Kurtz's voice instead.

"Sid, it's Bob."

"What is it?" I managed to say through the sudden chill I felt.

"Bad news. Her LDH is up again. Do you want to tell her, or should I?"

"How high is it? Wait, I think you should tell her."

I took the phone to Andrea on the deck, where she was sitting next to the pool looking at the ocean. "It's Bob," I said.

"Bob?" She took off her wide-brimmed sun hat to hold the phone against her ear, and the sun on her face showed her frowning. I hovered, watching her expression freeze in shock. Time and the wind and the ocean all stopped, sound stopped, and we were suspended in a moment of awful revelation. She turned to me slowly, her mouth moved, and the words thudded like boots in the night. "He says my LDH is back above six hundred."

The phone clattered on the deck. I knelt and held her. She sagged against me. Moments later, she roused herself. "I'm going for a walk. Come with me, Sid."

She changed in a fury to shorts, T-shirt, and sneakers. As we were exiting the house Daniel came up from the beach to get a bottle of water. She brushed by him. "What's wrong?" he said.

"Friday's blood test turned out bad," I said, and then went after her. I had to jog to catch her. She walked faster than she ever had before. I caught up, and fell in beside her. "Damn," she said. "Damn, damn, damn." We walked for ten minutes before she exploded again. "Damn." Otherwise there was just the sound of our breathing and our footsteps, and the surf smashing on the beach with the regularity of a funeral bell.

We rounded a corner of one of the streets and suddenly there were Joanna, Jonathan, and Daniel, waiting. Andrea didn't slow down. "I have to do this," she said. None of them said a word. They let us pass, and fell in behind us. We all walked around Amagansett following Andrea's fast pace. As we walked, the sound of their footfalls and their breathing felt like the advance of a supporting army. Their solidarity embraced me, lifted me so that even in that awful moment I felt we would survive in our togetherness. We walked for a long time as Andrea tried to exhaust her disappointment.

Home again, sweaty and spent, we fell into chairs around the big round table on the deck. Andrea looked around the table at the kids. "I guess you heard."

Jonathan — he was red-eyed from crying, as was Joanna — spoke for them all when he said, "Mom, just let us know whatever we can do." I ached for words that would make a difference, but could find none. Like Jonathan, I tried to let her know I was there for anything she needed.

What was there to say, after all? We had used up our best cards. After doing everything humanly possible to beat the cancer, it was back howling on our doorstep. I didn't know what to say, or what to do next. I had only hope. It told me we would find something, but I had no idea what options were left to explore.

I woke before dawn the next morning, when we would have to drive back to the city. Leaving Andrea asleep and Daisy curled on the foot of the bed, I put on shorts and a sweatshirt and walked barefoot onto the beach. The sand was cool under my feet. I walked to the water's edge. The waves were slow and heavy, they seemed to collapse in discouragement and dribbled up the sand. I turned to the dawn. To the east, the sky was fiery copper streaked with gray. A beautiful day was beginning.

"Why, God?" I asked. "Tell me why?"

Back in the city, Andrea's next CT scan confirmed the cancer's return.

DR. ROBINS had no strong suggestions. There were other kinds of chemotherapy, but the year bought by the cisplatin and the carboplatin that preceded the bone marrow transplant had come at great cost. Her bone marrow was worn out and could not take much heavy chemotherapy.

Dr. Casper suggested VP-16, taken orally rather than intravenously. The drug had a history of working in oral form with patients who had not responded to it intravenously. At the very least, if it would inhibit the division of the cancer cells and slow down the cancer's resurgence, it might buy us time to find another course. It was easier to take orally, but it was still toxic, and would still cause nausea and hair loss, and drop her white count, leaving her vulnerable to infections.

We were back where we had been last summer, except that this time, Andrea swallowed the drugs. Afterward, for the two days while the chemo laid her low with nausea and fatigue, she lay on the living room sofa. I stayed home with her, and we read the Bible together, or we held hands and meditated. She returned to some of the early meditations, trying to open her body to the medicine so it would be effective, and to find a restful and beautiful place away from the cancer. She told me that instead of imagining a beautiful place, she now thought back to Positano, and Provence, and to the little girl in Carcassonne. Her hair fell out again, and she dusted off her wigs. And as before, I kept an eye on the computer for the blood test results to be posted.

Amazingly, the tumor in Andrea's liver responded to the new therapy. The response was fast and dramatic. By August, her LDH was back down to 160. Her CT scans were clear again, the spots of tumor disappeared. Once more, we allowed ourselves to hope.

"Could this be it at last, oral VP-16 in small doses?" she asked after Bob Kurtz had reported the results of the latest blood test in which her LDH remained around 160.

"It looks good, doesn't it?"

"Let's hope it is," she said. "Maybe that's the best we can do."

Hope is a fire that never goes out, and flares up at the slightest encouragement.

Soon after Labor Day, she developed a cold that quickly got worse. X-rays showed she had pneumonia. We met with Bob Kurtz and Fry

Casper together in Bob's office. "I'm afraid it's the VP-16," Dr. Casper said. "Your bone marrow's not back all the way, and the drug's making it hard for you to manufacture white cells. You don't have any resistance. We're going to have to take you off of it."

Andrea, weak and fevered from the pneumonia, didn't argue. Without the VP-16, the tumor reasserted itself as quickly as it had disappeared. Her pneumonia cleared up in November, but when she started on the VP-16 again, the cancer cells were resistant and this time it had no effect.

Thanksgiving at the Steinbergs' was a different affair than it had been the year before. It wasn't grim on the surface; we treasured their company and their whole family too much for that. But the possibilities ahead of us were fewer, and we didn't know what to anticipate.

Chapter

27

I STOPPED checking the LDH figures at the end of November. They fluctuated wildly, down, then up again, as Fry Casper tried different kinds of chemotherapy. They were too discouraging, and we wanted to turn our minds to positive things. We had been married twenty-five years in December. Twenty-five years together, and to the casual eye we were blessed with the material comforts of an affluent life. In the last three years we had learned that time well spent with loved ones, caring time, attentive time, is the greatest and most precious blessing of them all.

My sister Hinda wanted to throw an anniversary party, but Andrea declined. She said she didn't want anybody to go to any trouble. Instead, we flew to San Juan, Puerto Rico, to celebrate our anniversary. Our hotel on the beach in Dorado, west of San Juan proper, was by chance celebrating its thirty-fifth year. Fireworks lit the sky in commemoration and sprinkled down to meet their reflections in the water; we watched from the terrace of our room and made the fireworks our own.

As they faded she leaned to me and whispered, "Happy anniversary, Sid."

How I loved it when she said my name, even after all that time. It wasn't any beauty in the name that moved me. In anybody else's voice, it would not have been the same. It was her mouth forming the sound, my name, the feeling it implied, that thrilled me as much twenty-five years after we were married as on the night we met.

Andrea kept an upbeat mood. The day's pleasures were enough. We walked and talked together on the beach and the hotel's miles of hiking trails, ate and drank, watched sunsets and made love, renewing our past honeymoons. We held hands at dinner, the ocean spotlighted outside the window, and she asked the mariachi band to play "We Wish You a Merry Christmas." We sat facing each other on the king-size bed in our room, closed our eyes, and meditated on an existence beyond the one we knew. Energy flowed between us. Our time was precious. We were realistic, but we kept the harsh truth in the background. We had learned to live on our emotional roller coaster, and for those few days we managed to wring joy from our moments.

Hanukkah, the eight-day festival of lights, began on December 9, and was bearing down when we returned to New York. Andrea plunged into planning the first of a series of family get-togethers. Hinda and her husband, Norbert, a Catholic, traditionally celebrated both Hanukkah and Christmas with their kids. This year, Andrea wanted to have them in the city. When they arrived from Princeton, I went to mass with Norbert. It was easy to recognize the Christian promise of salvation from the New Testament readings Andrea and I had done.

At home, Andrea set out potato latkes and applesauce, customary Hanukkah fare, on the coffee table. After Norbert and I returned from church, we lit the shammas, the candle used to light all the others, and then the first of the daily candles. Hanukkah commemorates the victory of Judah the Maccabee over the Syrian Greeks under Antiochus IV, and the reconsecration of the Temple in Jerusalem, and I recited in Hebrew, from memory, a brief blessing that could not have been more appropriate — it celebrated the miracles, deliverance, powerful deeds, and acts of salvation performed by God at this season. Then we moved to the dining room for Christmas dinner. Our prayers echoed both traditions

— our adherence to a belief in God, acceptance of the plan God had for us, everlasting hope, anticipation of a transforming afterlife.

The kids were around throughout the holidays. We had a wonderful Christmas dinner together. We felt close and free of tension, as if the issues between us had all dissolved. The feeling dated to that dramatic morning on the beach last summer, when they walked with us after Andrea got the news of her relapse. They were less like our children than friends, friends who wanted to be with us, and we with them. We enjoyed one another's company in a different and more mature way.

I ate during the holidays without restraint. I had stopped exercising, too, except for the walks I took with Andrea. Her relapse apparently had triggered a mild depression that sapped my self-discipline. I started gaining weight.

Andrea and I attended Pat Kadvan's New Year's Eve party, the third now since Andrea's symptoms woke her in the middle of the night. A friend of Pat's videotaped each party, actually, he taped the end of each year and the beginning of the next. He started with cityscapes from his apartment window while it was still light on December 31. He panned up to the sky, zoomed out past the waters of the East River to the Triborough Bridge in the distance. This is what it looked like, he was saying, as the old year gave up the ghost. Later, he focused on the party, and the guests.

Andrea and I arrived late, judging from the tape that I saw later. Nothing about us at first glance looked unusual. I was wearing a sport jacket and tie; Andrea wore a smart black dress and a wig, because her hair was gone from repeated salvos of chemotherapy. We took plates from the buffet and sat down side by side in straight chairs, held the plates on our laps, ate and talked with the others in the room. Andrea paid attention, as she always did, to the people around her. The quality of her attention, which distinguished her as a person with concern for others, was undiminished.

The clock rolled on to midnight. The champagne corks popped, and we toasted the arrival of another year. Welcoming 1994, we celebrated beating the odds for three years.

It was when the tape showed us leaving that I noticed what we had been working to avoid. I saw in myself, and in Andrea, an air of distraction, a kind of fatalism that made us more earnest, more cheerful than we needed to be. We were acting. We were denying.

AFTER the holidays, we continued a round of unsuccessful treatments. Fry Casper, consulting with Ian Robins and Bob Kurtz, tried ten different kinds of chemotherapy on Andrea. It wasn't that many, but that's what it seemed. Nothing worked for more than two or three weeks. The drugs killed more hair than cancer cells. She was bald, nauseated, and debilitated from the drugs, and there was no remission, no upside. Hope became harder to find, but still we looked.

Andrea's willingness to believe fully that she would be cured, a belief that held nothing back and left no cushion for disappointment, had departed with her first recurrence. After that, she adopted a tough realism. She was willing to hope, but not surrender to full-fledged belief. As one treatment failed and the next was offered, she demanded straightforward assessments of the odds.

"Don't give me empty promises," she said.

I had learned not to reassure her falsely. She wanted total honesty, no smiles or pats on the back, just the hard facts, without sugar coating. Since her first relapse and our night together at Carmine's, she told me and the kids, and all her doctors, consistently, "I don't want to be disappointed again."

As the VP-16 and now successive treatments failed, I knew more than ever how important was this form of self-protection. The string of disappointments was almost too much for me to bear. I still wanted her to be happy, healthy, contented, and at peace, enjoying all the goodness life can offer. My marriage vows said I would protect her. But I could not protect myself from disappointment.

Andrea, I think — we did not talk about it — now kept a place inside herself where death was a reality. Death, almost always somebody else's problem, had come home. I was emotionally bombarded, whipped like a leaf in a storm. I could not see to the other side of the hole her death would leave in my life.

Andrea was more realistic.

FRY Casper came into my office one day in January. Fry was young, with a kind, open face; Andrea liked him very much, to the extent of shopping for him and presenting him with a boldly colored sweater that he wore despite its contrasting with his more conservative, Brooks Brothers style. He took a chair across from my desk and looked me in the eye.

"Sid, this is hard to say," he began. "You know there's no longer any question of a cure. We're in a holding action. All we're accomplishing with Andrea now is palliation for a while. That's the most we can do."

I stared back at him, my mind swimming and drowning and trying to grab something to keep me afloat. "Why are you telling me this?" I blurted.

"She asked me to. She's afraid you may not understand. I said you did, but she wanted to be sure. We're talking months at best."

I thanked him for telling me, and when he left I sat rooted to my chair thinking, It cannot be over. It cannot be finished. There must be more than temporary relief in the cards.

"In the cards" was Andrea's expression. She knew. She accepted what I could not. When we talked about us, and the kids, our lives, she talked about now and tomorrow, not the distant future. That, she told me, "is not in the cards."

"What do you mean it's not in the cards. You just get dealt a hand of cards and that is it? You work with your cards. You play your hand the best you can." My protests were whispers in the wind, because in the end, what you're dealt is what you have to work with. You can make the most of it, but you can't get new cards.

"It's not in the cards, and that's the truth," she said. "It makes me sad. I think about my life, how I was brought up, what I wanted and couldn't have. I worked hard, Sid, you know I did. I wanted us to work, and we did, and I wanted our kids to be great kids, and they are, they're great people. That's a lot that I think I've accomplished. But to enjoy it for a long time, for us to take a long walk into the sunset, that's not in the cards."

I HAD held to my decision not to return to Casper Schmidt alone. I didn't think I needed to. The closeness I had achieved with Andrea, and the falling barriers between me and the kids, signified the strides I had made in the way I handled my relationships. But with Andrea's relapse, we again visited the psychiatrist together. We hoped that he might have some new treatment to suggest. Jonathan was the other member of the family who had continued seeing him from time to time to sort out his insecurities.

I had not seen Schmidt for several months when we made another joint appointment in the late winter. Andrea's diminishing options were preying on our minds. We thought, again, that he might have a new suggestion. We were reaching the point where we were almost willing to try anything.

Schmidt rang us into the building. When he opened the door to admit us to his consulting room, I had to fight to conceal my shock. He had lost weight dramatically. He had always been slender, but now his face was gaunt and skull-like, and his clothes hung from his frame.

There was only one logical answer, and it made everything fall into place. Suddenly, his expertise about cutting-edge cancer treatments like hyperthermia, his knowledge of immunotherapy with such drugs as interferon and DHEA, knowing who would prescribe them or where they could be found, his intimacy with the details of white blood cell counts, the fact that he had been able to offer Andrea his own DHEA capsules, all made sense. Schmidt had AIDS. It wasn't his patients', it was his own disease that had driven him to acquire so much knowledge. I don't know why I hadn't suspected it before. I remembered Robins's telling me that Schmidt had first approached him as a member of ACT UP.

"Are you okay? You've lost a lot of weight," I said. Suddenly the concerns we had come to talk about seemed less important.

"Fine, thank you. Shall we begin?"

He obviously didn't want to talk about his problems, and throughout the session he gave no hint that anything was wrong. I didn't feel comfortable pressing him. But another answer was unlikely. I understood that he was carrying a burden as great as Andrea's, but it seemed strange that he'd done nothing to let his patients know.

I thought how odd it was that he knew the most intimate details of our lives, but we knew almost nothing about his. He had been married once, I thought, but maybe it was only an impression. The primary feeling given by his offices, and the private apartment I had glimpsed occasionally behind his waiting room, was of nonattachment, a life that seemed purely intellectual.

He knew of no new weapons that we could add to our arsenal, he said. He told Andrea to stick to her diet, her vitamin supplements, and her DHEA. "Some new drug may still show up," he said. "Some combinations are proving effective. Anything can happen."

But he spoke with an air of resignation.

"He has AIDS," I said to Andrea as we drove back across town in light Saturday traffic.

"I think so, too."

"Why didn't you say anything?"

"I don't know. It didn't seem important, I mean, not to our relationship. He's dying, too, like me. It's why he knows so much, and seems to care so much about what I'm going through."

"Do you think that's why he was so hard on you?" I said.

"I think he wants me to get it right. He knew we didn't have all the time in the world."

But questions echoed through my mind. Serious, disturbing questions. I remembered Schmidt's appearance on a local cable show called *Fifty Minutes;* the panel was talking about the psychological factors driving politics, and Schmidt was among the most vociferous in claiming that politicians acted mostly to meet psychological, not social, needs.

I remembered, too, seeing a monograph he'd written arguing that AIDS was a manifestation of guilt feelings. Gay AIDS sufferers, he said, were expressing their guilt over being homosexual to the rest of the world through a process of self-selection — by selecting themselves as victims. Schmidt not only had embraced the plague metaphor for AIDS, the disease as a judgment on society, but had made it psychologically self-inflicted. His silence made sense in that context, as another expression of guilt, and his guilt must have been colossal.

His exhortations of Andrea also made sense. It was critical for him to get her to succeed in controlling her illness. That would provide living proof of the individual's ability to control with her mind a disease that was ravaging the body. It would give him hope and strengthen his resolve.

And at the end, when Andrea had relapsed and his own body was giving up its resistance, he was ashamed. He had lost the battle. He could not do for himself what he was urging and telling his patients they could do. His theories were a house of cards, and he was the proof of it. He could not prepare his patients for his absence because he could not admit that he had AIDS. The loss of power was too great to accept.

Andrea indeed had been a mirror in which Schmidt tried and hoped to see himself. He was the White Knight who had driven her to new heights of self-empowerment, who had demanded that she find within herself the resources to fight her battle. But he also was the Black Knight, trapped by his own diagnosis, who played out his life's destiny through her. She was a foil for his mortality, and she danced to the tune played by his demons.

A few weeks later, on a Sunday, I waited in the car with my coffee and the paper while Andrea met with Schmidt. I was finishing the Arts and Leisure section when she opened the car door and announced grimly, "He's not seeing patients anymore." There was desperation in her voice. "He gave me the name of another therapist."

By coincidence, we were meeting Jonathan for brunch at a restaurant on Broadway. Andrea told him Dr. Schmidt was going to stop seeing patients. Jonathan said he was not surprised. Recalling a session months earlier, he said, "I was describing the behavior of one of my professors, and Dr. Schmidt got this look on his face. It was a peaceful look that seemed amused and tolerant of the things of this world. It struck me as the look of someone looking back at life. I told a friend of mine, who knows him, that I had the sense that he was dying."

Andrea, however, could not release Schmidt from her life. Her need for his approval was too great. "I know he's sick, but I can't see another therapist," she said. "I'm not going through the whole thing with anybody else. I can't, and I won't."

Without telling me beforehand, she went to his office unannounced. That night, she told me in a shaken voice what had happened.

The doctor had answered the door in his bathrobe. He was more emaciated and obviously ill. "What do you want?" he had demanded, angry at the disruption of his privacy.

"I want to see you. I need to ask you some questions."

"I don't feel well, as you can see. As I told everyone, I'm not seeing patients, even when they show up on my doorstep, and I can't answer any questions."

"But I just need . . ."

"I'm sorry, but you'll have to go." He had closed the door in her face.

Andrea was shaken for days afterward. Schmidt's inability to ward off the onset of his own disease stole her confidence and increased her sense of vulnerability. If Dr. Schmidt, with all he knew, could not prevail, what hope was there for her?

But eventually she felt relief. The fact that Schmidt could not save himself by the powers of his mind lifted a great burden; she no longer had to control her destiny alone. She could attack the cancer medically, without the fear that her psychological state would undermine whatever new therapy she tried. This, in an odd way, gave her confidence that she could handle her latest battle on her own.

She was free at last from the myth of the cancer personality, free from the metaphor that defined cancer as a stealthy invader seeking out susceptible, and thus guilty, individuals.

Chapter

28

IAN ROBINS and Fry Casper still had some options up their
sleeves. There were still drugs that Andrea had not tried, and some
new ones that had just come out.

Ian said, "When protocols don't work, sometimes you just take
something off the shelf and use it and you may see a miracle."

We still were hoping for that miracle. Andrea, demanding realism
on the one hand, strived to maintain her optimism on the other. She
kept a tiny yellow notebook at her bedside. In it, she drew a misshapen
blob under which she wrote, "The only cancer that you will ever need."
But as successive chemotherapies failed, her need for hope drew us into
a spiderweb.

So far, Andrea had followed cutting-edge but sound treatments,
administered under prescribed medical conditions. She had added
self-empowering complementary medicine in her blend of relaxation
techniques, stress reduction, nutrition, and exercise. The vitamin supplements and DHEA she took, even the now-discontinued interferon
and somatostatin and the herbs, were in addition to, not instead of,
the treatments that conventional doctors in the mainstream of cancer

treatment had prescribed. Now she began to grasp at straws. The snake oil peddlers of the cancer treatment world made sure plenty were available.

Here, too, I followed Andrea's wish that I help her.

I started collecting, at her request, articles that described the most miraculous cures. We read together profiles of doctors who cured their patients with detoxification routines after conventional therapies failed. My folders of research began to bulge with recipes for "liver flushes" of apple juice, Epsom salts, olive oil, and phosphoric acid; "clean sweep" protocols of fiber in the form of psyllium seed husks and clay in suspension designed to plow stored wastes from the intestines; purges triggered by two-day juice fasts of citrus juice, Epsom salts, and water. We read instructions for coffee enemas, oil soaks, salt and soda baths, mustard foot soaks, and castor oil compresses, all designed to rid the body of "toxins, wastes, and byproducts of tumor breakdown."

I wrote letters, and arranged telephone consultations with people whose concern oozed through the phone. Thus came the conversation with the enzyme capsule man who told Andrea her blood urea nitrogen was "slightly off" when I knew it was normal, and proposed his enzyme capsules as the answer. And a suggestion that she take nutritional supplements totaling hundreds of pills daily. And a description of footbaths that would cure everything from epilepsy to cancer. And also a nine-page letter from an alternative medicine clearinghouse in Washington State that began, "If I were in your shoes, I would eschew conventional therapy and look for a systemic therapy that has a track record of success on a broad spectrum of neoplasms."

The writer went on to describe, in impressive medical jargon, programs in Japan, Sweden, and the Bahamas, clinics in Canada and Germany, and a number of other treatments he suggested offered Andrea some promise. Among the dizzying array of options this "consultation" produced were an "herbal soup" created by a pharmacologist, and a mixture of herbs, vitamins, beans, garlic, ginger, scallions, and other ingredients costing $125 a bottle.

I don't doubt the writer was sincere. He wrote that most conventional cancer doctors "are working from the same cookbook, and what we need is a larger, new cookbook with greater flexibility and greater concern for individual needs." Hurrah for that!

All the same, his letter to Andrea angered me with its sly digs at conventional medicine's inability to offer her a cure. He touted a therapy of which he wrote, "Unfortunately, this is a therapy that is not administered anywhere in the United States. To which many doctors will pooh-pooh and say, as so many do at your husband's institution, 'Anything they can do there, we can do here.' No so. Take my word for it."

Trust me. The peddlers of the extreme and untested alternative therapies about which Andrea and I read all seemed to have one thing in common. They held out their particular approach as her only hope, and said, "Trust me."

In the absence of clinical trials proving their claims, there is little else for the advocates — often the salespeople and profiteers — of such therapies to say. That is the essence of their appeal. Like a deathbed conversion, they offer the hope of last-minute salvation. They take advantage of frustration and fear.

I had become a believer in nonconventional aspects of medicine since Andrea enlisted me. That is, I believed in complementary medicine that integrated conventional therapy with a range of adjunctive treatments. I had seen the value to her of believing and actively participating in conventional treatment programs, of following her spiritual beliefs, of stress reduction and relaxation techniques such as meditation, and appropriate exercise and diet. Other approaches she had followed, such as vitamin supplements and herbs, and drugs like interferon, somatostatin, and DHEA, needed further evaluation, but I had learned not to dismiss alternatives with potential. I saw that they can form, with conventional cancer treatments, a holistic attack on the disease. Many "alternative" medicine practitioners actually practice complementary medicine. As Bernie Siegel says of his meditations, "They can be used in conjunction with all other supports, including the medical profession, and your spiritual resources."

Complementary or integrative medicine does not reject conventional therapy. It does not disparage reputable treatment centers, or try to convince patients that wonder cures await if they will follow the Pied

Piper. It is extreme alternative medicine, quasi-medicine on the fringes, that lures desperate people with promises of results that no other treatments can hope to match.

Andrea and I understood that level of desperation now.

A S we contemplated ever more radical approaches, many small miracles kept us going. One was the miracle of friendship. Dr. Judy Fineberg, Andrea's friend from Atlanta, arrived in March for a visit. For several days, they were like college roommates again, shopping, attending movies, prowling museums, and laughing at almost every turn.

It seemed to me, watching from afar as I had when we were in Atlanta, that their best fun was the simplest. I would leave for the hospital with the two of them sitting over coffee and bagels at the kitchen table, and they might be there again when I returned.

"It's amazing," Judy said one night when the three of us were out for dinner. Andrea had gone to the bathroom. "She's just like she was in college. Something strikes her funny, and she leans back and laughs the same laugh, the one I remember from college days, her larynx bobbing up and down.

"You know, she had me meditate with her," Judy added. "We sat together, and we held hands and gazed into each other's eyes, and she played a meditation tape you had made for her."

I had made a couple of the tapes, when we first started exploring the possibilities of meditation. I had read them to her, one on taking medicine within and another on the pain patients share with others, and because she liked my voice she had wanted them on tape for times when I couldn't be there to read them to her. Both were my own variations of meditations she had discovered. The one she had listened to with Judy asked that "we share the pain of others, and they share ours, so that together we can heal our wounds and ease our pain and overcome our suffering."

"It really seemed good for her," Judy said. "She said it always made her a lot calmer."

The next night, before Judy was to leave the following morning, they were dressing to go to a book club discussion when I heard them burst into laughter. Andrea, bald from the successive rounds of chemo, had put on her makeup and false eyelashes and then one of her wigs before she turned to her friend and said, "Not bad, huh?" as if they were heading out for a blind date.

Andrea was in a cancer support group at that time. In the group, the patients spoke of three-month goals, the kinds of goals I encouraged my patients to aim for when an anniversary or a child's wedding was coming up. Judy was leaving to return to Atlanta when Andrea said, "I'm going to set a three-month goal that you'll come back in May and we'll celebrate our birthdays together." Judy's birthday followed Andrea's by nine days.

"Why not set a six-month goal?" Judy enthused.

Andrea smiled quietly and said, "Let's just set a three-month goal for now."

PASSOVER fell at the end of March. Andrea's sister and her family came from New Jersey for the first-night seder, which Andrea had organized at home despite fatigue and a low blood count from chemotherapy. Marsha, six years older, had escaped the emotional turmoil that Andrea brought from her childhood, but she sympathized with her younger sister. Our apartment was full with the two of us, Daniel, Joanna, and Jonathan, Marsha and Bruce, their sons David and Lawrence, Lawrence's wife, Donna, and their new baby, and David's fiancée, Sylvia.

Andrea gathered up the child with love. "No, no, no," she protested, unleashing her wonderful laugh. "I'm too young to be a great-aunt."

On Passover's second night, we returned with Daniel and Jonathan to my sister Joyce's for the seder we had attended almost every year.

When it was over, Jonathan drove back to Manhattan with Daniel in the front seat while Andrea slept, exhausted, in the back seat beside me. I suddenly realized that, beginning with the Hanukkah-Christmas party with Hinda and Norbert in December, she had organized a kind of farewell tour. The round of dinners, including each branch of the family, provided ceremonies at which to say goodbye, without facing the finality.

WE clung to our routines, trying to keep the framework of normalcy together. One day in April, as the weather had begun to soften, we went out together for a walk around the neighborhood. Andrea was wearing tights, a sweatshirt, and her baseball cap. We were just strolling. She couldn't walk faster, but I should have been. Starting with the year-end holidays, I had been getting no exercise, and when I sat down at the table I seemed to have no discipline. My waist had ballooned. I was pushing a hundred and ninety pounds, too much for my five-foot, ten-inch frame. I felt heavy and out of shape, but I couldn't think of focusing on myself now. Andrea needed all my attention. Suddenly she jabbed me in the ribs and said, "Look."

Across the street, where she was pointing, a white-haired couple was walking hand-in-hand. As we watched, the man nuzzled the woman's neck and, to my amazement, she squeezed his bottom under his tweed jacket.

We once had talked about growing old together, walking down the streets with nowhere particular to go, holding hands. We imagined that our days would take us into coffee shops, to museums and concerts, or maybe we would just stay home and read and listen to music in the living room. We would enjoy our children, welcome them and their families to our apartment, bounce grandchildren on our knees. That was the old age we foresaw, and every time Andrea saw an older couple holding hands she'd point them out to me. "There we are in twenty years," she would say.

Now she said, "I used to think that would be us. Remember?"

ANDREA, unsuccessful at seeing Dr. Schmidt, continued to call him. Eventually, her calls went unanswered. Her need for his guidance was replaced by concern for his health.

"He's sick, Sid," she told me. "You have to find him. Even if he can't talk to me, he ought to know we care."

I tracked him down at St. Vincent's, one of the hospitals in the city with a large AIDS treatment program. The Patient Information operator put my call through to his room.

Dr. Schmidt responded gruffly when I identified myself. Andrea picked up the extension and said, "It's Andrea. Is there anything we can do?"

"Nothing. It's better if you don't call me," he said. Then he softened. "I'm sorry. We spent many years in psychotherapy together, the whole point of which was to leave you on your own. Now that has happened. You'll have to go it alone without me from here on in."

"Did you try mop therapy?" she said.

"Mop therapy? Oh, yes." He recalled her visualization of men with mops and pails scrubbing her liver. Visualization and guided imagery were never part of his therapeutic arsenal. "Maybe I should try it," he said gently.

"Can we help you? Is there anything we can do?" Andrea repeated.

"No, thank you," he said wearily. "I have to help myself, and you have your own fight. But I'm confident that you can do it. You deserve to win. Remember that. You are Andrea, the deserving person, the wonderful mother, the deserving wife. That's the main thing to remember. Now please, do me a favor and don't call me again."

Andrea hung up the phone with tears in her eyes. They didn't speak again.

Chapter

29

I F I have to die, will it be painful?"

As one chemotherapy drug after another failed, death haunted Andrea and she started asking me this question. So far all of her treatments had produced relatively little discomfort and few side effects. She had weathered them all well and come through in good spirits, even the violent "shake and bake" response to the antifungal drug administered to wipe out her blood infection. She was concerned — we both were — with maintaining a good quality of life even in the face of death. She wanted to die painlessly.

"No," I told her. "If you die, your liver will fail, and you'll just go to sleep."

I didn't anticipate her final series of treatments.

At this point, with each successive drug, she wanted reassurance. She would ask me, as we lay in bed at night, "Sid, feel my liver, will you? Is it any smaller? Is this drug working."

I would feel her abdomen. Her liver was rock hard, full of tumor, and I felt numb as I lied, "Yes, I think it's a little smaller."

"She's asking me to feel her liver. She wants me to tell her it's smaller, but it's not," I told Bob Kurtz and Fry Casper, when I couldn't stand the deception and the terrible sick feeling I got each time.

They were shocked. "You're not her doctor," Fry said.

"I know, but . . ."

"But don't do it. It's not fair of her to ask you. You can't tell her the truth, and it's emotionally devastating. It's going to kill you if you continue. You have to stop now."

The last of the chemotherapies failed. There was nothing left to try. We had discussed liver transplantation earlier, but that was not an option because her liver continued to receive cancer cells from the lymphatic system. Then Bob Kurtz suggested one last-ditch effort, a treatment we had talked about but put off in favor of the different chemos.

"It's a desperate measure at this point," Bob said. "But if she has a good response, it can give her another period of life, a little more time."

What Bob wanted to do was block the blood flow to the portion of Andrea's liver that contained the tumor mass in a procedure called hepatic artery embolization. The lack of nourishment kills the proliferating cancer cells, and normal cells as well. It's done by inserting a catheter into the hepatic artery and introducing tiny sterile balls called pledgets. The arterial blood flow carries them along into successively smaller blood vessels until they can't go any farther. Picture a golf ball stuck in a hose — the water can't get through no matter how high the pressure gets.

Fry was against it. "It's more likely to hurt than help," he said. "Liver embolizations cause infections, severe pain, liver failure, fever. Is that what she wants at this point?"

Two philosophies were at work. Both were valid, and not mutually exclusive. Good medicine means, as Bob proposed, giving people the options and letting them choose. It also means, as Fry argued, finding a balance between side effects and therapeutic effects.

It was up to Andrea. She wanted to try it. Time was running out. Her LDH had climbed to astronomical levels — 3,500. The prior elevations, by comparison, were child's play.

Dr. Botet at Memorial Sloan-Kettering performed the procedure. Studies of embolization showed it normally works better for the indolent type of tumor, but Andrea's response at first was encouraging. A CT scan showed the procedure had killed off a lot of tumor.

It also, inevitably, killed off a lot of normal tissue. The damage to her healthy liver cells produced side effects more debilitating than any she had suffered. She weakened physically. She developed an ileus, a paralysis of intestinal activity. Nothing moved in her intestines. Gas trapped there swelled her belly until she looked as if she were nine months pregnant.

I began to give her enemas, regular enemas at first to get her bowels moving. When they didn't work, she requested coffee enemas. I ground fresh beans, brewed the coffee in diluted form, let it cool, and then prepared and administered the enema. We did this every morning. Alternative medicine claims coffee enemas remove toxins from the large intestine and prevent them from reaching the liver through circulation. Andrea simply wanted to reduce her distension. She so badly wanted them to work, but nothing really changed. Nothing worked. She was uncomfortable and miserable.

The embolization's effectiveness at killing cancer cells, however, prompted Bob to suggest a second one, blocking blood flow to another portion of the liver.

Fry, opposed to the first embolization, was even more reluctant. "We don't have anything left, but I don't want to make her sicker and more uncomfortable," he said.

They approached her again. She still had not fully recovered from the effects of the first embolization. As they talked, I could see in her face, for the first time in the three and a half years since her tumor was discovered, that she knew it probably wouldn't work. She believed not only that it would not help her, but that there was a good chance it would increase her misery. She saw the suggestion for what it was, a desperate, last-minute maneuver when there was nothing left to try.

But she agreed to go ahead, even though she wasn't physically or mentally ready, and afterward, her fears were realized. The ileus worsened. Combined with the necrosis in her liver — the death of normal as well as cancer cells — her sickness and discomfort worsened.

I knew she thought if she could just ride through the discomfort, it would pass like a big wave. I believed it, too. I had to. We would get through this just like we had gotten through everything else the last three and a half years had thrown at us, from the moment we thought she had just months to live. She still survived. We had always found a way somehow.

I STOPPED working in May, after the second embolization. Andrea was home from the hospital, and I wanted to spend as much time with her as I could. She celebrated her forty-ninth birthday on May 6. Two days later, Mother's Day arrived. She remained swollen and uncomfortable. I ground beans, brewed coffee, let it cool, and administered an enema. She sighed and shook her head; nothing moved. I went out for bagels. On the streets families wearing church clothes held hands and carried shiny balloons vividly marked with red hearts and "Mom." Daniel and Jonathan had told us to expect them later. Joanna was still in Madison, nearing the end of her sophomore year.

Andrea moved with difficulty into the living room. She sank onto the sofa and groaned. "This is what I didn't want," she said. "I didn't want it to ever be like this."

Daisy jumped up and nestled at her side as I brought Mother's Day cards for her to open. Two Miró lithographs hung behind her on the wall. I had looked at them for years, but now the surrealist's blotches and swirls, full of color and energy and movement, seemed sinister to me, Andrea's disease in abstract. She read the cards and passed them to me. The children had chosen cards with sentimental rhymes, to which they'd added messages. They amounted to valedictories. They were trying hard not to say goodbye, but what they had written sounded final.

Joanna's card read, "I think we have . . . a very wonderful and special relationship. You are and will always be in my heart. I know you're working as hard as you can and I hope one day I'll be as strong as you are. I love you more than you know, Mom."

Jonathan thanked his mother for the many lessons she conveyed to him. "You have been teaching me things since I was two and you taught me arithmetic, but most of all you have taught me simply to love a lot and to be a good person. That's the most important thing I have learned from anyone."

Daniel wrote from his deep empathy with Andrea, from all those times when he had elected himself her stand-in as my emotional sparring partner. "I don't think that I've ever really told you just how much you mean to me," he had written. "You are the wonderful special person in my life. You've always been there for me, in my heart and in my thoughts. I love you more than anything."

I, too, had written a card that said, with its undertone of finality, perhaps more than it needed to say. I assured Andrea that my love for her would grow ever stronger, and signed it, "Your husband forever."

She rose and moved slowly to the grand piano, where she arranged the cards on its closed top. "They're good kids, aren't they, Sid?" she said. "We did do a good job, didn't we?"

"You did," I said.

"Joanna is terrific," she continued as she moved back to the sofa. It was painful to watch her, her grace stolen by the congestion in her system. "She works hard, she's responsible. Her instincts are on target, so you just listen to her when she tells you what she wants to do, just encourage her to do her own thing and ask the right questions and let her instincts do the rest. She'll know what's right, all you have to do is help point the way. Do that, and she'll soar."

I listened knowing she was transferring responsibility to me. But I really had nothing else to do. Joanna was almost twenty, nearing the end of her second year in college. Jonathan was completing his third year at Columbia. Daniel had moved into the full-time undergraduate program at NYU, where he was studying political science. The nurturing, the lessons, the shaping had been done, and Andrea had done the most of it. My job, I thought, was to remember my own hard-earned lessons, and to be the father I had worked hard to be.

"Enjoy and share Daniel's sense of humor," Andrea said. She was reclining on the sofa, smiling. "I know we poke fun at you sometimes, Sid, but it's just when you're too serious. He's smart, he has style, but you have to keep your feet on the ground when he tells you things. He's a flatterer, you know.

"With Jonathan, listen to his intellect. You'll know him through his poetry, and the books he reads. He'll tell you everything through that, but you'll have to listen, truly listen.

"They're going to be fine," she said. "I'm so proud of them. You be there for them, if they need you, Sid. But don't go to them. I always tried to be too big a part of them. It's better to let them come to you."

"I will, I will." I knelt beside her and buried my face in the crevice of her neck, as if hiding from the prospect of parenthood without her. I couldn't take her place. No matter that the children were grown and accomplished, there would always be an empty place from their mother dying young. I remembered when my mother met Andrea, how I craved her approval and, when she gave it, how proud and glad I was. Daniel and Jonathan would miss that. And I sensed that the bond between Andrea and Joanna, already strong, would have enriched and deepened over time. Those things I could never give our children.

MAY wound toward June. Andrea moved awkwardly about the apartment, and we took slow walks around the neighborhood. I kept giving her the coffee enemas, hoping they would give her some relief. Eventually, she felt well enough to ride out to Amagansett for a weekend.

Daniel went with us. When he was a teenager, he had invited hordes of his friends for beach weekends; they gave us no peace and ate us out of house and home. When we finally understood that it was our right to say no, or to tell him to invite one or two friends and not six, the problem ended. This weekend, there was no question of bringing friends. It was private. We all knew, though no one said it, that it was the last time we would be together at a place we loved.

We went out to Montauk for an early dinner at Gosman's Dock, one of our favorite dining places. Before we ate, we walked onto the beach and took some pictures. Andrea wore a bright dress, and a straw hat to cover her baldness. Nobody looking would have seen anything but a family recording a light moment. When we sat down, Andrea stared out the window at the fishing boats. She looked all around, as if she was trying to fix the place in her mind. Afterward, she and Daniel spoke quietly for a long time while I walked along the docks.

"What did you talk about?" I asked Daniel later. We had gone out to the beach, bundled in sweaters against the cool night. Andrea, exhausted, had gone to bed.

"It wasn't what she said. She was looking at me with a kind of envy. I know she was thinking I was strong and healthy and she wasn't." He stopped to tug a fisherman's cork and a shred of net out of the sand. "Then she said, 'It's all beautiful, isn't it? It's sad that I'm not going to be here after a while.'"

We walked along in silence. After a time Daniel added, "She was almost apologetic that she wasn't going to be around. She was worried about us missing her."

The wind blew. Something, maybe it was sand, stung my eyes and blurred the way.

Her premonition showed in the pictures we had taken on the beach when they came back from the photo shop. The sadness of goodbye was in her dark eyes looking at the camera.

JONATHAN ended his year at Columbia and moved from his dorm back to the apartment. He announced that he was thinking of taking a summer course in ancient Greek at City University. A tutor was helping him get ready. Soon he was going around with his head buried in three-by-five-inch notecards. Andrea was impressed, as she always had been by intellectual achievement.

"Do you want to walk with me, Jonathan?" she asked one day as he was poring over his cards.

He looked up, and there was none of the reluctance to be with her that had distressed her when she talked with Dr. Schmidt the year before. He just smiled and said, "Let's go."

She pushed herself up from the sofa, put on a Columbia sweatshirt in his honor and one of her baseball caps, and they headed to the elevator. I watched from the terrace as they moved slowly down the street. Jonathan was glancing at his cards as they moved out of sight behind a building.

They came back after a long time, and Andrea fell asleep. "We walked a good mile today," Jonathan reported. "I don't know whether it was being with me, or getting some exercise, or being outside, but she really liked it. It meant a lot to her. She has a lot of strength. I didn't think she could go on such long walks."

"It was being with you," I said. "She admires you. She admires your intelligence. It must be the index cards and the fact that you're learning ancient Greek."

Jonathan looked proud.

They walked frequently after that. She tried to take one walk every day. More than that was difficult, and she spent the rest of the time on the sofa. At night, sleep came hard. Often I woke to find her struggling out of bed to move into the living room. She said the sofa was more comfortable. It was painful to watch her, but she wanted to think she was letting me sleep. I hardly recognized her shuffling shape. Each step was labor.

She was in pain, but she refused to take medication for it because she preferred to be alert.

I read to her when we were together in the living room. I enjoyed it, and I suppose I was pleased that she liked the sound of my voice. What she wanted now was the Bible, as I did. We returned over and over to our favorite passages from the Song of Songs that so vividly expressed our love for one another. But increasingly she wanted to hear about the trials of Jesus. I read from Matthew and Mark, and she hung on the descriptions of Jesus's suffering. What she hoped to find was equanimity in suffering, a way of bearing it with understanding.

Ian Robins, his wife, and son were in New York at the beginning of June, and came by the apartment. Andrea dressed for the occasion. Her abdomen was distended with loops of air-filled bowel, and she was uncomfortable, but she put on makeup and a colorful turban. Robins spent some time with her alone.

"If I can buy some time, I'll buy it," she told him. "But if I'm going to die, I'm going to die."

He told me later, when Andrea was talking with Floriane and Amani, that he thought it was rare that she still cared about how she looked.

"You can help patients to accept their death, or accept the fact that they're going to die," he said. "But I don't think they fully accept it, they get resigned to it. A true acceptance of death is really rare. If they're resigned, they don't care how they look. But look at her.

"You know, I've been impressed with her attitude right from the beginning. I wondered what she got in psychotherapy that did it. I have to tell you, I don't think I've ever had a more involved relationship with a patient. I had to fight to keep from losing my perspective. You're lucky, Sid. She's one of the most together and complete women that I've ever met."

"He likes you," I told Andrea when they had left.

She smiled. "I told him that people who believe in life after death are more likely to be accepting, rather than resigned. Nobody wants to go into another life looking like a schlump."

THE days seemed alternately to speed and drag. They dragged when she was restless or uncomfortable. At least then, I was conscious of my time with her. Sometimes I looked up from the Bible I'd been reading to see the windows dark and wondered how another day had gone without my knowing it.

Word reached us that Casper Schmidt had died. We both were shaken. My ambivalence about his methods in Andrea's psychotherapy, and my initial aversion to the therapies he suggested for her cancer, had been overcome by my feeling that he had genuinely cared. The alternative or complementary therapies to which he introduced Andrea gave her hope. They had given us both hope, and hope was a great component of the miracle of these last years. As a therapist, he was her anti-parent, and she was as anguished by his death as she had been at both her mother's and her father's.

I believed, in the end, that he truly loved Andrea professionally and did everything in his power to save her and to lead her to self-empowerment. He had acted like a classic Freudian, saying little in their sessions, until she got sick. It was only then that he pushed her toward treatment options and became more confrontational in urging her to resolve her underlying conflicts. He felt they faced a common enemy, and he guided her in ways that he felt would help them both. I was sorry he felt such a great measure of guilt and the great burden of feeling he had to cure himself. Andrea, in her fight, improved her quality of life. I hoped he did as well, for he loved books and music and was an artist, and I hoped he had a companion who loved him as much as I loved Andrea.

She still felt angry, in those last days, that her parents were not there as she was dying. She felt that at the moment of her greatest need they had abandoned her again. It still upset her that her mother had outlived her by twenty-six years. It seemed to Andrea the ultimate unfairness.

Joanna remained in Wisconsin as Andrea's days dwindled. She was finishing her spring semester, and Andrea wanted her left alone. "Don't call her home. Let her finish her finals and get through the year. It's too soon, anyway."

This was not just about exams. Andrea still felt guilty about abandoning Joanna, and she wanted to protect every step Joanna took toward independence. She didn't want to compromise that independence by calling her back home.

I was torn, wanting to satisfy Andrea's wish yet not wanting Joanna to feel excluded. Ultimately, I thought Andrea needed the satisfaction and that Joanna was strong enough to understand her mother's wish.

"She was like totally dying when I was taking my finals," Joanna said later, "and I didn't know. I mean, I knew, and I was throwing myself into my books like I had never done before."

She had planned to stay on in Madison for a week following her finals, but her brothers called her home. Daniel called first. He said it was his duty as her brother to tell her what was going on and that she needed to come home.

"Why didn't they tell me?" she cried indignantly.

Jonathan called Joanna the next day. He told her it was only fair that Andrea see her while she still was able, mentally and physically, to appreciate her children's company.

The week after Joanna arrived, Andrea, to everyone's astonishment, got off the couch, got dressed, and took her shopping. Joanna saw the shopping expedition as a final chance to give Andrea a portrait of her as a grown daughter.

"It was her pride and joy," Joanna said. "She had a vision of how she wanted me to look. She wanted to visualize me in nice clothes. I mean, she could barely walk, and there she was taking me to Banana Republic."

Andrea didn't go out after that. She stayed at home, and Joanna read to her from *Jonathan Livingston Seagull.* It quickly became one of Andrea's favorites, especially a passage near the end:

"But then the day came that Chiang vanished. He had been talking quietly with them all, exhorting them never to stop their learning and their practicing and their striving to understand more of the perfect invisible principle of all life. Then, as he spoke, his feathers went brighter and brighter and at last turned so brilliant that no gull could look upon him.

" 'Jonathan,' he said, and these were the last words that he spoke, 'Keep working on love.'

"When they could see again, Chiang was gone."

Chapter

30

A N D R E A entered the hospital a few days later. Still swollen and uncomfortable, feeling the effects of the blockage in her bowel from the embolization, she expected to go home again. She arranged with the physical therapist who was working with her to visit her at home, and she told relatives and friends who wanted to visit not to come.

"The death watch is starting," she said, after I told her that my sister Hinda had called to say she was coming to the city to be with us.

Andrea wanted none of it. She wanted no wringing hands and halting sentences set off by awkward silences. Her playful spirit refused to allow it. She wanted laughter and to remember things we had all enjoyed.

"Tell her not to come today," she said.

She already had resisted Judy Fineberg, her friend for almost thirty years, who had helped see us through that first experiment with interferon, accompanied her on a trip to Madison, and meditated with her in March. Judy had called, but Andrea told her to stay home. "I'm a mess," she said. "I'd love to see you, but not like this. Wait till I'm home again."

Her hope lived on. But on a Wednesday night, everything changed.

Blood tests showed her liver had started to fail. It could no longer, with the kidneys, push fluid through her system. Instead of being excreted as urine, the fluid leaked into her tissues, adding to the water that was already there normally. She started to swell. Her skin stretched as the tissues beneath expanded. At the same time, she was enormously thirsty. She begged for water and drank constantly, but no amount of water could satisfy her thirst. Her body grew larger and larger, no longer from trapped gas, but from the water in her tissues her body could not excrete.

At the end of the second week of June, there was no reason to pretend she was not dying. I acknowledged this for the first time. My denial until now of the fatal nature of her cancer had been essential for my hope, and hers.

"Do you want to come home?" I asked. We had convened a family council meeting in her room, with Joanna and Jonathan, her neurologist, and the head of the hospital's pain service.

The final decisions, as much as the first ones, were hers. She looked out at us from eyes buried behind swollen cheeks. "To tell the truth, the prospect of moving doesn't thrill me. I'm too uncomfortable. I think I'll just stay here."

She repeated her fear that she would die in pain. The neurologist encouraged her to take as much pain medication as she needed.

"You mean I don't have to have pain?" she said. "I don't have to suffer?"

"No, you don't."

Joanna turned away. I experienced one of those shocks of recognition. In a few days she would be gone.

But in the days ahead she used little of the morphine. She preferred a measure of pain to oblivion. She didn't like the feeling of not being clear. She wanted, even now, to be available to the kids and me.

Those days in June escape my memory. They might have been beautiful, as late spring days in New York can be, with flowers sprouting in window boxes and foliage greening the parks. Or they were dank like the June day two years earlier when Joanna graduated from high school. I don't know. We all rushed between Memorial Hospital and the apartment, and no ray of sunshine or drop of rain made the slightest difference. My existence was confined to her hospital room.

We talked a lot, all five of us. Nothing had to be said, but we had memories to savor. Andrea didn't really want anybody around. She wanted no death vigil, no pitying looks when she wasn't feeling or looking her best. But our need for her was great and she rose to the occasion. She rejected sadness and demanded laughter. With all attention riveted on her, she was a generous, tender, gracious star, recounting with the children details of their lives. It was a loving time. We held hands, we kissed, we hugged.

Andrea and I, when we were alone, talked about death. We had spoken of death many times. I knew she was more worried about how her loved ones would feel after she died than about dying.

She had wanted to hold on to her life on earth, because of its moments. Inevitably, the smallest moments, the ones people tend to overlook, grow large. At night, when our voices sometimes seemed to be the only thing holding off death's approach, we talked about the earthly moments Emily evoked in Thornton Wilder's *Our Town,* moments as common and rare and precious as the smell of fresh coffee brewing in the morning.

I saw in her acceptance of death the belief that she would transcend earthly existence and make a peaceful transition to a higher state. She had come to terms with her life on earth, with who she was, and with who or what she would be in the next life. She believed — as I do, as I must — that she would enter the realm of the spirits, a realm from which we all come and into which we all eventually move again through death.

"It's all right to move on," she told me. "When it's time, it's time. But I'll miss this life, with all of its 'ordinary' experiences. They don't seem ordinary anymore."

Once she was in her new existence, with guiding spirits to help her find her way, we would communicate again. I would speak to her, tell her about my life, the kids, the world that I could see and touch and feel. She would whisper to me words of love and convey the wisdom that came from her passage. She was serene in this belief, knowing she would leave a legacy of love as she entered a place of peace.

THE week drew to a close and Andrea seemed stable. Joanna and Daniel debated on Friday whether to go to the beach house for the weekend. Marsha and Bruce arrived, and Andrea and her sister said a tear-stained goodbye. Hinda came, and Andrea asked her to leave after fifteen minutes. Later Jonathan, recognizing that I was worn physically and mentally, volunteered to spell me sitting through the night with Andrea. "You've been here every night. You need a rest," he said.

He was right. I was at the limit of my resources. Staying at the hospital had allowed me precious time with Andrea, but I agreed to let him stay. Later, Daniel made the same offer. They agreed to split the duty; Daniel would stay on Friday night, Jonathan on Saturday.

Andrea was by now grotesquely swollen. She was, or seemed, twice her normal size. Her failing kidneys and liver continued to leak fluids from her vascular system into her tissues. She drank constantly without relief from thirst. She felt as if she had to urinate, but could not. But she was still an entity, a personage, a palpable human being. That is to say, I had no sense of her approaching absence, of there being a void where she now was.

I returned to her room on Saturday morning. Daniel rose from the couch where he had slept. Andrea was asleep. He whispered that she woke him four times during the night for water. He left for Wing Chun practice, not wanting to wake her to say goodbye. There would still be time, he thought.

A nurse came, got her up, and helped her to the bathroom. Andrea's each step was clearly torture; she moved as if hobbled by arthritis. The nurse made her bed with clean sheets and pillowcases. She struggled back, with me helping her this time, and sank into the bed again.

Her swollen hand found mine and her eyes pleaded. She said, "I don't want to move anymore."

She closed her eyes and lapsed into coma.

That afternoon, I made the necessary phone calls summoning the family. As at the beginning, when the cancer was discovered, I functioned on some vague robotic level. Marsha and Bruce were there, and Hinda and Joyce, but I was hardly aware of them. Daniel and Jonathan met outside the hospital and came to her room together. Joanna arrived red-eyed. The wait began.

We all were caught up in the storm of feelings that death causes. Emotions ricocheted like bullets. Death is hard to get right. You have only one chance, and it is such an awesome thing the way it plays on the emotions. Jonathan was bitter. There would be no tomorrow night for him to sit and talk with her. Joanna was angry, too. She would accuse me of not informing her how close her mother was to death. I think she knew, and did not want to face it any more than I did. My brain told me Andrea was dying even as my heart denied it. The deaths I had experienced in my life — my sister Rita when I was a boy, my parents, patients I had grown close to — were nothing as compared with this. I was miserable, and frightened of the void I saw ahead — walking, eating, sleeping, facing the world alone. Even as Andrea lay in her final coma, I could not imagine that she would not be there.

We waited. Night fell. Joanna left, returned, and left again to wait at the apartment, yearning for escape from the charged emotions of the moment. Marsha also went home to the apartment to be with Joanna. Bruce waited in the television lounge outside in the hall. Andrea's breath grew shallow. Jonathan and Daniel kissed her and told her they loved her. They gave me the final moments.

IN all my years of being a doctor, with all the patients that I had seen dying and taking their last breaths, none died with the tenderness and grace I saw in Andrea. But then, I had never watched so closely.

I was comforted to be with her. I whispered, "Andrea, Andrea, I'm here." Something in me knew that she could hear me, and I knew that being with her now was where I belonged. I was accompanying her as far as I could. Surely she sensed my presence at her side and drew from it the last solace I could give her.

I watched her every breath. I watched her lips, her mouth, her eyes, her face, and all of her expressions. I watched how life evaporated and removed its affect, influence, and driving force from all aspects of her body. Like an engine shutting down, her breathing slowed and stopped, her heart took one last beat, the warmth of her skin dissipated into the air, the color left her face, the small flutterings of eyes and lips and nostrils quieted, her body lost its tension, the grasp of her hand on mine relaxed.

I whispered my last words to her physical presence: "I love you. Your guiding spirits will help you. Speak to me from the other side. I'll be listening."

I have thought of this scene a thousand times, trying to project myself into the tunnel through which she approached the light and the spirits reaching out to guide her. I think of it less as time passes. Now the scenes my mind invites are the ones she whispers to me, scenes of Andrea alive, in all her beauty, her elegance, her wit, her humor, her smoky, lusty laugh, her warmth, her vitality and courage. I remember her as joy and energy, as movement and emotion, all those aspects that I believe survive in the realm she now inhabits.

Chapter

31

T HE world grinds on and respects nothing. We arrived at an Upper West Side funeral home to view the casket the night before the funeral. Suddenly, police cars roared into the streets around us with their sirens screaming. The air crackled with the sound of their radios. The cops jumped out and looked skyward. We followed their eyes and saw a man standing on a window ledge, high up. Another man — a counselor? — seemed to be pleading with him.

"That's considerate," my sister Joyce murmured. "If you're going to kill yourself, do it near a funeral home."

There were details that had to be attended to. Protocols. Paperwork. The body had to be identified. A check had to be written. I was in a daze. I kept looking for Andrea beside me.

The funeral was at noon the next day, June 21. It was Daniel's twenty-fourth birthday. He, Joanna, Jonathan, and I stood together in an anteroom at Temple Shaaray Tefila while more people than I thought I knew filed by, shaking our hands, hugging us, speaking words of condolence that I barely heard. I had the vague sense that Andrea was receiving a remarkable outpouring of affection. When we moved into the sanctuary, a place of worship converted from a movie theater, I was surprised to find it filled with several hundred people.

Rabbi Harvey Tattelbaum knew Andrea well. He encouraged the mourners to celebrate Andrea's "beautiful life," a life that "was a search for meaning. She left no medical, physical, or spiritual stone unturned. She fought with science and medication and mind. She rose to great levels of spirituality — a spirituality that made her draw her family close to her beyond words that could express such love and closeness.

"That in her life that was poetic, playful, delightful," the rabbi said, "must not be belied by the tragedy of her death at the age of forty-nine. The challenge to her survivors is to be resigned to the inexplicable, and in the midst of sorrow, perceive joy. A legacy — of courage, of beauty, of devotion — has been given you. Love each other more because of it. Take care of yourselves, and of each other. Take her spirit as a blessing, and love and help each other more. Your love for each other will be your greatest gift to her, and ultimately to yourselves as well."

Joanna had excused herself from speaking. Hinda would speak for the women in the family. Joanna sobbed and I held her hand while Daniel and Jonathan spoke in turn. Both spoke of things that Andrea found dear. Daniel extolled her love of laughter: "Even to the end and in great pain she kept her wonderful sense of humor. Of all the gifts that she gave me, what I will cherish most was her belief that life was meant to be enjoyed, and the playful way that she went about living it." Jonathan recalled his mother's love of the beauty of language: "She knew how much I loved her, yet every time I could express it to her in the lines of a poem that she loved, it was as if a mountain moved inside her, as if her life suddenly brightened."

Daniel put his finger on Andrea's greatest satisfaction, the one thing she had demanded of herself unremittingly. He spoke for all three children when he said, "She died believing that she had prepared us for our lives, and I believe that she did, and we will make her proud."

At last the mantle fell on me. I had worked almost obsessively on my remarks. In the few days since her death I had felt guilty, wondering if I had told her often and passionately enough how much I loved her.

Every word I had written said, "I love you," as if I had never said the words before.

I told the crowded sanctuary I wanted to speak as Andrea Winawer's husband, to celebrate her life. Then, knowing that every listener who had ever loved would understand, I spoke her praises. I quoted poems that revealed her playful spirit, her undying sense of youth. I read from the Song of Songs the passages that we had read to one another, that expressed the beauty of love, and the passage Joanna had read to her from *Jonathan Livingston Seagull*, on love's importance in all things. I recalled her life and her struggle, her courage, her commitment to me and the children.

"Andrea wanted you all to know that she was not defeated," I said. "On the contrary, she achieved her important life's goals and did not wish to be anyone else. She gave us everything she had, and what she had was remarkable. We have it now, and through us her spirit will remain, surrounding us with love, and through her strength we will have strength to go on and continue her work."

A final poem expressed my feelings the way my own words could not, and I read to the audience from Kahlil Gibran's *The Prophet*:

Farewell to you and the youth I have spent with you.
It was but yesterday we met in a dream.
You have sung to me in my aloneness, and I of your longings have built a
*   tower in the sky.*
But now our sleep has fled and our dream is over, and it is no longer dawn.
The noontide is upon us and our half waking has turned to fuller day, and
*   we must part.*
If in the twilight of memory we should meet once more, we shall speak again
*   together and you shall sing to me a deeper song.*
And if our hands should meet in another dream we shall build another
*   tower in the sky.*

"I will love you forever, my sweet Andrea."

I left the podium shaking and drained. As I sat down I saw my children were all holding hands. Behind them, people were exchanging glances, wiping eyes. What did they make of this emotional, sentimental, shattered man? I took comfort in the knowledge that the miracle of Andrea continued. It was not only in the past but in the future, living in the memory of her sweetness, innocence, and loving spirit.

W E sat shiva for three days. People came and went, my sisters, Andrea's sister, their children, our friends, the rabbi. The children and I shook many hands, were held in many arms. Food appeared on the table, was eaten, and the plates disappeared as if by magic. We all moved through the apartment like zombies.

Friday and the end of the traditional mourning period arrived. We went to temple for Friday evening's Shabbat service, and prayed together. Then we packed the car and prepared to drive out to Amagansett.

Joanna said, "It feels like we're packing our lives."

But the four of us, alone together without Andrea for the first time, still felt like a family. We were a family with a void, going through the motions, but in the movement it felt, surprisingly, as if we would survive. Family and friends came out to be with us. Their presence warmed us, but we needed the solitude of our own thoughts, the silence to let our feelings speak. We carried our grief in different ways.

I took long walks by myself on the beach. I spoke to Andrea, telling her how much I missed her. I looked at the sky and saw her spirit in the clouds. I heard her voice in the sounds of the seagulls.

Every evening as the sun went down I sat on the deck of the house and wrote to her. Every crash of the waves on the beach brought memories that surged and then disappeared into the sand. I wrote words of love that I imagined rising to her from the page — how wonderful and vital and soft and tender and sensitive she was. I poured out memories, wishes, and regrets. I wrote how desperately I missed her.

"Where are you? Oh, God, I can't bear it. I love you so much. It was all too short," I wrote. "I will come and visit you soon. I want to see if you are really there. Maybe it's some sort of cheap trick, a bad dream, and it's not really happening after all. I want to talk to you close, and be near you and feel your presence. We all do. I don't think I will ever be completely happy again."

I cried all the time. I was inconsolable.

Joanna, Jonathan, and Daniel grieved quietly in their own ways and moved on. The summer ended, and Joanna returned to college in Madison. Jonathan entered his senior year at Columbia. Daniel continued at NYU as a matriculating student. I put this news in my letters to Andrea. She would be glad to know the kids were doing fine.

Returning to the city, I haunted bookstores and scooped up every book in sight on grieving and loss, just as Andrea bought books on meditation, life after death, visualization, and whatever else she needed to help her. I needed these books to help me now. They all said the same thing, but that was okay, because that told me it was true. We who grieve go through stages.

I was in the first stage of shocked numbness. I read C. S. Lewis. He wrote about this stage that the shock is so great, the loss so enormous, it blurs everything. It blurred even my recollection of how Andrea looked. Photographs didn't help. I could not bear looking at them, anyway. They were painful, static, one-dimensional. They froze Andrea without capturing her movement and speech. The books helped. I joined a grieving group and met weekly with a grief counselor. This helped. Crying my heart out on the beach and yelling at the ocean, cursing the waves, this helped. I yelled at God, demanding answers. None came back, but it helped, anyway. Family and friends helped. Even talking to Andrea's dog, Daisy, helped; at least she looked back at me with moist Yorkie eyes and seemed to understand I was pleading. We both missed her, after all.

The kids helped most of all. Without them, and the perspective I maintained by thinking about them, I might have walked into the waves.

I visited the cemetery, the grave that would not bear a marker until the anniversary of her burial. I felt close to her, and talked to her, but I could not stand doing this for long, and each time I left after a few minutes.

The letters helped me release my grief. I wrote them compulsively, every night for six months. Then I stopped. Suddenly, almost overnight, it seemed, I didn't want to write another letter or read another grieving book. I still talked to Andrea, and listened for her voice. I felt her presence. I felt it so strongly, almost as if she had touched me, that sometimes I would turn around to see if she was there, and for a fleeting second I would see her image. She appeared to me clearly again. Her voice formed out of the void and spoke to me. "Listen to the kids," she said. "I love you. Talk to me." I heard and felt her love, felt her transmitting it to me almost as if she had taken me to her bosom and embraced me.

The shock had worn off, but the emptiness remained. She was with me, and yet not with me. The effect was monumental. I never had known such profound loss, never knew what it was, but I was moving on. I knew I was moving into the second stage of grieving.

I reentered the world. Andrea had wanted me not to be alone. I went on dates. I would sit with them, talking over coffee, but after an hour or so I would start comparing them to her and I would have to say goodnight. I went to the opera by myself and cried. If I found myself alone in the evening, I went out to a movie in the neighborhood. I could not stay home except to sleep, and now, for the first time, sleep did not come easily. It came only with fatigue, and even then, I was up after a few hours.

I began to reach out to friends. Some old friends were there for me, some were not. I found new ones, and I reached out to family more than I ever did before. My social life, my connections, my activities were entirely in my hands for the first time. Without Andrea to make arrangements, I had to make the phone calls and make the plans.

I found it helped to have a plan. Giving myself a goal to move toward instead of drifting provided peace, comfort, and a feeling of security as I put my life back together. My plan for surviving loss often included reaching out to friends and family. It included travel, exercise, and reading books. It included whatever worked.

Fortunately, I had a foundation to build on. I am basically a social person; I like people, love the opera and physical activities like biking, skiing, and working out at the gym. I began to pursue activities like these. I began to nurture myself. In my new life, I even learned how to shop in a supermarket.

As time went on, I was no less affected by Andrea's death. But I saw more clearly the healing lessons of her life, her illness, her optimism, and her courage. Using her lessons, I continued the process of transformation that I had begun with her. Her lessons grew large to me, and I embraced them fully in my practice and my life.

Epilogue

HEALING
LESSONS

I LOOK back over the three and a half years of Andrea's illness with a mixture of feelings and conclusions. I believe with all my heart that Andrea chose the right path for herself and for us as a family, and for me as a spouse. Her choices — primarily the choice of self-empowerment — extended her life, I am convinced, from months to years. I have no doubt of that.

The quality of her life and of our lives together was tremendously enhanced to a degree I never would have thought possible. It is sad that it took cancer to make us live our lives more fully. What a compounded tragedy it would have been not to recognize and use its onset as the opportunity it was to demand more of ourselves and to love each other better.

Recently, rummaging in some old things, I came across Andrea's junior high school yearbook. I was startled to find her described as someone who "looks upon adversity as opportunity." Perhaps, at the tender age of junior high school graduation, she was trying to reconcile not being allowed to attend the High School of Performing Arts and was looking for opportunity in her disappointment. But I was impressed by the consistency of her philosophy. Strengths that go unrecognized often surface in adversity.

Until her illness I failed to appreciate how strong Andrea was. It was her strength of will and the power of her belief in her choices that pulled me into the world of complementary and alternative medicine. At first, I was torn between my love for her and my devotion to the conventional medicine I knew and had always practiced. Love won, and I ended up convinced that mainstream medicine must ultimately embrace the lessons to which she exposed me.

I'm glad I followed her along this path. It opened up new medical vistas to me. I did the right thing for her, and for my own role in medicine. It comforts me and will always comfort me that I used my medical resources to help her, without letting blind adherence to convention get in the way. She always knew she could count on me. She told me so early on, when we were still dating, in a poem she called "What Is a Sidney Jerome?"

> *He is a blue and gold bathrobe* [she wrote]
> *with sometimes white thongs.*
> *He is a tiny sweet baby*
> *needing love and affection and tender care,*
> *for he is fragile.*
>
> *He is a man, my man,*
> *whom I need so desperately because*
> *he understands.*
> *He is a man with character and wisdom*
> *and gentleness.*
>
> *He is a voice on the telephone*
> *lilting, resonant, always saying*
> *the right thing.*
> *On a cold night when it's hard to sleep*
> *he is a warm body, always ready*
> *to hold and cuddle.*

He is a man with a heart
and unselfishness
who wants to share,
never shutting me out.
Waiting for the right moment
to tell me things.

He is a man giving me love
and a reason to be living.

What strikes me as I read it now is her excitement about me and our relationship. How grateful I am for that. How grateful I am that she knew I would be there for her always.

Having someone to count on when you're in need is a blessing and so important in a battle, but being there for someone is not to do things for them that will take away their self-empowerment. The companion in the battle must support independence and self-help. The key is to provide support without turning it into something smothering that creates dependence, inactivity, self-pity, and depression. Those things will de-power a relationship and lessen the quality of life.

We physicians have always been trained to keep people alive. Anything else is a failure. We as doctors and the medical establishment have to get over that. Of course survival is monumental, but death is not a failure. We all die. Not living is the failure. Patients who embrace life, whether they survive or succumb, will, as Larry LeShan puts it, "live the fullest."

Andrea and I lived the fullest. My joining her battle brought us closer together. Reading from the Bible, saying prayers, sharing books, our walks and talks, talking about our most hidden and deepest desires, fears, concerns, and beliefs, raised our union to levels of spirituality and intimacy I had not known we could achieve. Our experience reordered our priorities. We had wanted to grow old together, to linger over coffee, walk the dog, enjoy our children and their children. We wanted to be that white-haired couple walking down the street and holding hands, while people smiled to see us. What we learned was not to wait. We learned to take the moments that were given us.

I had never known such a union as I had with Andrea. I don't know if it will ever happen to me again, but it is possible. To have had such a blessing once is a rare thing, and if it comes along again I will feel doubly blessed. Andrea would want that, as she told me many times before she died. Such a rare experience requires a special emotional and spiritual connection between two people who are ready, able, and willing to make it happen. It took Andrea and me over twenty years and the challenge of cancer, but the remarkable thing is that it did happen.

My relationship to the children changed dramatically. Without them I would have fallen off the face of the earth when Andrea died. I always had cherished them. With her illness and death, I cherished them more and felt an urgency in our relationships. The facets of each sparkled more brightly and clearly in my eyes. Each is an individual, but our common ground lies in our love for Andrea and for each other. Each carries an outstanding set of human values. I listen to them more carefully now because I must. I am the only one.

I know what they need from me now. I understand it and I see it clearly. They need me to be there, they need me to validate their feelings, their instincts, to hear of their accomplishments and of their problems. They use me as a sounding board to allow them to make their own choices, to find their own directions, to solve their own problems. They need me not to tell them what to do, but to help them in any way they wish me to help. My role is to nurture, to reinforce their own responses to inner feelings and instincts, and to help them see the larger picture in their lives when they are faced with decisions. They all know what to do, they all have direction, they all have what it takes. I am totally and completely happy and satisfied with them and take great pride in each one of them. I love them immensely and deeply, and they know it. I have told them so many times, as I told Andrea and as she told me. Whatever they do and whatever they need I will be totally in support of them.

Where do I go from here? I want to go farther on the path Andrea and I walked together. In Andrea's absence, without the challenge that I helped her face, I sometimes wonder if I can move ahead. I realize that I don't know the answers. But I have learned enough to ask the questions and to make changes.

How can I continue to improve myself personally? How can I be a better man, a better father? How can I carve out a place where I can be generous in offering, graceful in receiving, wise in understanding, and laugh a lot along the way? How can I pluck moments from the rush of time?

I continue to believe I will meet up with Andrea again one day. I continue to believe in the light at the end of the tunnel and hands that will guide me to another life. When that day comes, I will tell her about myself, about Joanna, and Jonathan, and Daniel, about our families, our friends, about life in her beloved New York. I will tell her that we were guided by the inscription on her gravestone, "May Her Love Remain With Us," and that we felt her love.

I still feel it in those moments when she speaks to me and I turn around thinking for a second she is there. She is so close I can almost touch her. I know in my heart that one day the energy of our souls will entwine again somewhere in the universe and that, once again, we will build our citadel of love as we move through endless universes never, finally, to be parted.

Until then, in my professional life, I am busier than ever. I see more patients, do more endoscopic procedures, conduct more research, write, and lecture more throughout the country and the world. I feel that I am on a mission.

Part of it is to preach the gospel of cancer prevention, primarily in colon cancer, based on my vision, my understanding of the disease, the evidence generated by twenty-five years of research and my analysis of research elsewhere. This one cancer accounts for 135,000 new cases among men and women and more than 50,000 deaths in the United States alone each year. We can reduce this death toll by more than half with the screening techniques and the lifestyle modifications that are available today. I chaired an independent multidisciplinary panel that for two years examined all the evidence related to colon cancer screening and concluded that every man and woman in this country over the age of fifty should be screened for colon cancer. Screening for colon cancer is as effective — and cost-effective — as screening for breast cancer with mammography.

Women especially should care about colon cancer screening. The incidence and mortality of colon cancer among women is much higher than that of cancer of the cervix, for which women screen routinely with Pap smears. It approaches that for breast cancer, for which mammographic screening is now accepted and routine. A good lifestyle, which includes a diet low in fat and high in fruits and vegetables, abstinence from cigarette smoking, a reasonable body weight, and a reduction of alcohol intake to a minimum, can further reduce the incidence and mortality from this disease.

I published these conclusions on behalf of our panel in a peer-reviewed journal in 1997. It was received exceptionally well throughout the world as the definitive, evidence-based, state-of-the-art analysis and set of guidelines for preventing colon cancer. I worked closely with the American Cancer Society, which developed guidelines using ours as a resource, and as director for the World Health Organization's Center for the Prevention of Colon Cancer at Memorial Sloan-Kettering. One result was new Medicare guidelines, effective at the beginning of 1998, that allows reimbursement of people for cancer screening. This change in public policy will benefit many, and I feel professional satisfaction in my role in the research and advocacy that made it happen.

After Andrea's death, I wrote a book, *Cancer Free,* with my good friend and colleague Dr. Moshe Shike, on the prevention of all cancers. This book, published in 1995, is written for the public, easy to read, user-friendly, and stocked full of the latest information on lifestyle, diet, environmental factors, alcohol, smoking, genetics, and screening for all known preventable cancers. It has been estimated by the National Cancer Institute that if all available measures were adopted nationwide we could reduce the death toll from cancer in this country by one half.

Today half a million people die from cancer every year in the United States. I personally believe that prevention holds an important key to further progress in cancer control.

My own personal research in colon cancer has now turned to the uncovering of susceptibility, especially genetic susceptibility. I published, in collaboration with colleagues at my institution and at New York University and Johns Hopkins, a paper demonstrating a new inherited genetic mutation in Ashkenazi Jews that places them at increased risk for colon cancer. We are embarking on further studies in this area. If we can identify people in the general population who are susceptible to cancer, we can then target our preventive strategies in an efficient and cost-effective manner to reduce their risks. The bad news, when we have a positive genetic test, is that these individuals have an increased risk. The good news is that we can do something about it. We can offer colonoscopies, in which a long fiber optic–lighted tube is used to examine the entire colon. Premalignant polyps then can be removed. A large multicenter trial called the National Polyp Study, which I led, demonstrated that removing premalignant benign growths reduces the chance of getting colon cancer by 90 percent.

I have expanded my horizons in cancer prevention to encompass not only greater efforts in colon cancer but also a major focus on cancer in general. In addition to publishing *Cancer Free,* I have been offered, and have accepted, the chair of the Cancer Prevention and Control Program at Memorial Sloan-Kettering. This is a huge challenge. It means bringing together all the investigators and clinicians interested in cancer prevention and control at our institution, dealing with inpatients and outpatients and facilities at the main campus and in new diagnostic and wellness centers that we have recently developed. It ranges as far as new centers with community hospitals in areas outside New York City, including New Jersey, Westchester County, and Long Island. This is a far-reaching program that involves molecular biology, behavioral science, nutrition, and lifestyle changes, epidemiology, genetics, psychiatry, and the new area of chemoprevention — the prevention of cancer by the use of drugs and dietary supplements, including vitamins and food extracts. This new challenge has taken me into collaborative efforts with other institutions that have similar interests, such as M. D. Anderson in Texas, the Fox Chase Cancer Center in Philadelphia, and the American Health Foundation in New York City.

Identifying susceptibility in people and offering them lifestyle modifications, screening for the early detection of cancer before it becomes lethal, and uncovering benign growths such as polyps before they become cancerous are keys to the next major set of advances in the control of cancer. This will be the next breakthrough, saving hundreds of thousands of lives each year.

As a result of my experience with Andrea I learned quite a bit about complementary and alternative medicine. However, I feel I have only just scratched the surface and have a long way to go.

Conventional or mainstream medicine has set the standards for the diagnosis and treatment of disease since the mid-1880s. However, in recent years, consumer trust in conventional medicine has eroded and large numbers of Americans now seek complementary and alternative medicine that is considered to be outside conventional medicine. A survey conducted by Dr. David Eisenberg in Boston found that 61 million Americans used some form of complementary or alternative medicine, and 22 million saw one of its practitioners for a medical problem. The magnitude of this trend is reflected in the $14 billion a year estimated to be spent by Americans alone on alternative treatments.

In recognition of the importance of these forms of medicine, the U.S. Congress in 1991 appropriated $2 million to establish an Office of Complementary and Alternative Medicine at the National Institutes of Health. Its aim has been to more adequately explore this area. This office held a series of workshops beginning in 1992 to help develop a database of research and practices, and provided support for ten complementary and alternative medicine centers in the United States. It has been designated as a World Health Organization Collaborating Center in Traditional Medicine. The word "traditional" is used to indicate methods that existed prior to modern medicine.

Further recognition of the consumer demand and possible health benefits of complementary and alternative medicine has been made by health maintenance organizations. An Oxford Health Plan survey revealed that one in three members reported visiting a complementary or alternative practitioner, a pattern being seen in most of the large HMOs. Oxford, serving 1.5 million people, has provided member access to practitioners, including acupuncturists, massage therapists, chiropractors, dieticians, and mind-body healers. At this writing, Oxford planned to expand its pool of these practitioners, and to send its forty thousand member physicians to courses on incorporating complementary and alternative methods.

Patients with cancer use complementary or alternative therapies frequently, and have for some time. In a survey conducted at the Cancer Research Center of Hawaii in 1984, 50 percent of the patients reported some use of alternative therapies, and another 8 percent said they used them exclusively. The therapies used included prayer, herbs, vitamins, nutrition, and psychological methods.

This all raises critical issues. We in conventional medicine need to understand why patients seek complementary and alternative treatments, so that we can modify our approaches to be more responsive to their needs. We need to learn more about possible adverse interactions, not to deny patients access to complementary and alternative treatments, but to make sure patients benefit. Finally, we need to explore the entire field for new and effective approaches to treating cancer, which could improve quality of life and alter outcome. We have to remember that many highly effective medical procedures now in the mainstream were once considered to be unconventional. Radiation therapy has such a history. It also is well known that many effective drugs in common use had their origin in herbs that were used as part of traditional medicine.

Although the literature of complementary and alternative medicine abounds with claims of effectiveness, studies are generally of poor quality and the evidence weak. Some well-designed studies have been conducted but are not readily available from on-line databases or have not been translated into English. Such studies generally are not published in the usual scientific journals. There is a need for experienced investigators to examine the merit of promising complementary and alternative approaches, and to publish their findings in readily accessible, peer-reviewed journals for wide dissemination and critique. The NIH Office of Complementary and Alternative Medicine has taken steps toward developing a system for identifying promising practices and encouraging their scientific assessment.

As the foremost cancer center worldwide, Memorial Sloan-Kettering must lead in investigating and attempting to understand these areas. We must learn what nonconventional practices cancer patients are engaged in and determine how these could affect their treatment and outcome. We must understand why cancer patients are turning to these forms of medicine. We must inform cancer patients about appropriate complementary and alternative medicine options from our credible perspective and provide guidance based on scientific inquiry and analysis of available evidence. Patients with cancer often are in shock from their diagnosis. They are likely to be bewildered by barrages of hard-to-interpret information. We can do a better job of helping them sort through what's available. Finally, Memorial Sloan-Kettering must take a leadership role in the scientific investigation of any promising approaches for the control of cancer, whether it be in the areas of conventional treatment, prevention and wellness, or complementary and alternative medicine.

The distinctions between conventional and other forms of medicine are not always clear. Complementary medicine and alternative medicine are generally considered to be practices that are not widely taught in conventional U.S. medical schools or adopted clinically in hospitals. They are "patient centered" rather than "physician centered." They focus on stimulating the patient's ability to fight on his own behalf in order to enhance the natural healing process. Complementary medicine is a relatively recent term indicating that the unconventional therapy is used as an *adjunct* to conventional medicine. Andrea's use of immuno-stimulants, including herbs, to stimulate the immune system during her conventional cancer treatment is an example.

Alternative medicine, on the other hand, implies *exclusive* use of an approach that is unconventional. The term "integrative medicine" has been used by Dr. Andrew Weil and others as a substitute for "complementary and alternative medicine." They point out that integrative medicine pulls together many approaches that are considered to be part of conventional medicine but perhaps not used widely, such as nutritional guidance and stress reduction techniques. I agree that the term "integrative medicine" may better define this growing field, which combines the best of conventional, complementary, and alternative medicine.

There are many reasons why conventional medicine views these areas with some suspicion despite their rising popularity. One is the tendency of some practitioners and advocates to steer patients away from conventional treatments. Another is the many claims of effectiveness without scientifically established proof. Alternative medicine sometimes uses seemingly bizarre diagnostic methods. Some practitioners will say they can detect wind going through the kidneys as evidence of kidney disease. There are unfamiliar treatments like detoxification. For these reasons, an atmosphere of confrontation between conventional and alternative medicine has arisen.

I believe we must resist confrontation. Each has something to offer the patient, which after all is our main concern. It doesn't matter where progress is made as long as it is the truth. Conventional medicine has made great strides through the scientific process and can provide the expertise through which progress can be made in promising complementary methods. We at Memorial Sloan-Kettering are in a unique position in that regard. We have the expertise to properly evaluate promising methods of prevention, diagnosis, and treatment, whatever their source.

Since Andrea's death my knowledge of complementary and alternative medicine has expanded. Recently I have attended seminars and meetings at the National Institutes of Health and at Columbia University medical school. I have talked to many of the major practitioners of complementary and alternative medicine in this country and elsewhere. I have developed working relationships with the complementary and alternative medicine centers at the University of Texas, at the NIH, and

at the Rosenthal Center at Presbyterian Hospital in New York, and with
Dr. Weil's program at the University of Arizona. I will also serve on the
editorial board of Dr. Weil's journal, *Integrative Medicine.* I have begun
to integrate many aspects of complementary medicine into my own
practice. I now ask patients about their use of complementary medicine. I am able to offer guidance about aspects that I know about, especially nutrition, physical exercise, and relaxation techniques such as
meditation and visualization.

As I write this, I have been asked to develop an integrative medicine
program at Memorial Sloan-Kettering. This would be a great step for
the field and for our hospital. In preparation for this challenge, I have
started inquiries at our center and have been impressed, but not surprised, at the level of patient interest. Many services already are in place
on an individual basis. For example, our patient librarian told me that
almost five thousand patients checked out meditation tapes over a five-
year period. Thousands of others have taken out books on meditation
and other aspects of complementary medicine, especially in the mind-
body area. Individuals at our center already are engaged in art therapy,
meditation, and visualization.

Complementary and alternative medicine is quite far-ranging. It includes not only nutrition and mind-body intervention, but also phar-
macological and biological treatments, herbal medicine, and
bioelectromagnetics. This is the detection of electromagnetic wave disturbances in the body for diagnosis and the use of electrical stimulation
for bone healing and the location of acupuncture points. Entire systems
of alternative medical practice have been developed. We need to determine, through scientific study, which therapies from this vast array offer genuine promise, so we can put them to work for the benefit of
patients.

Many medicines today, for example, have their origins in herbs.
Herbs are used by 10 percent of the U.S. population. The Food and
Drug Administration has recognized their potential value and now per-
mits animal studies and pilot clinical trials to further evaluate them.
The FDA further understands that while for some herbs the active

ingredient has been identified, for others it has not, and has agreed to permit testing of the whole herb rather than individual constituents. Herbs have been used for many disorders, including cancer, and have been the origin of some very powerful chemotherapeutic drugs such as vincristine (periwinkle) and Taxol (bark of the yew tree). Well-known herbs in use today include ginkgo, Saint-John's-wort, ginseng, and garlic. However, the quality, efficacy, and method of extraction of herbal products can vary widely among producers and even from batch to batch from the same producer. They can be contaminated with bacteria, fungi, and trace metals. Some herbs can even be deadly, such as pokeweed, which can cause vomiting and bleeding.

In some European countries, herbs are treated as drugs to be dispensed only by a physician's prescription, and they are used widely there. In Germany, for example, Saint-John's-wort is more commonly prescribed than Prozac for depression and is said to be as effective.

Very little is as yet known about the effectiveness of these herbs in treating cancer, and little is known about their adverse interactions with chemotherapeutic drugs, antibiotics, and radiation therapy. But we certainly need to investigate them and keep an open mind.

Andrea sought out complementary medicine. She did not dismiss conventional medicine but developed her own integrated system of complementary and conventional medicine that she felt was to her best advantage. I believe that this improved our quality of life and our relationship immensely and probably improved and lengthened her survival. I cannot prove this, of course. It is my gut feeling, knowing the natural history and aggressiveness of her cancer and how long she survived with it, and knowing the beautiful quality of life that she had in spite of her diagnosis. The benefits were obvious, whether it was the methods she incorporated in her treatment, or the personality that gave her an advantage in the first place when facing adversity. Or maybe it was yet another factor, a resilient biological system centered in her immune system or another aspect of her physiology. Perhaps it was because she took very little in the way of drugs all her life that her system was exquisitely sensitive to her treatment.

This latter concept is an important one. We can intervene in our biology very easily, perhaps too easily. We have learned from infectious diseases that when we treat frequently with antibiotics, resistant organisms can appear that are more difficult to control. We know in cancer that when we kill off the cells that are responsive there are other cells that are less responsive or unresponsive to the treatment that grow wildly, producing recurrences and ultimately death. There is much that we do not know.

Research in conventional medicine has one goal that is certainly in common with complementary medicine. That is the search for new and promising approaches that will break through the frontiers of present knowledge. I have learned many things through my experience with Andrea in the past few years and since, but the major lesson is to keep learning and to keep an open mind. This is the best way to assure progress in anything, including the control of one of mankind's most lethal enemies.

Andrea helped bring hyperthermia a giant step closer to becoming accepted cancer therapy. Through her treatment in Wisconsin and my discussions about it with many people at Sloan-Kettering, Dr. Lloyd Old became interested in it. Dr. Old, the world-renowned immunologist at Sloan-Kettering, is also the medical director of the Ludwig Institute and the Cancer Research Institute, the latter organized by Dr. William Coley's daughter, Dr. Helen Coley-Naughts. CRI has funded cancer research primarily in the field of immunology. Because of Dr. Coley's work in stimulating, with a fever-producing bacterial toxin, the immune system in cancer patients, the institute expressed an interest in Ian Robins's hyperthermia and its effects on the immune system. The institute has supported his research, helped obtain patents on his unit, and placed several hyperthermia units around the world for collaborative research with Dr. Robins. All this because of Andrea. Who knows what miracles may yet be brought to patients with cancer as a result of Andrea's search for new methods? Hyperthermia was once considered outside the mainstream of medicine. In the future it may provide us with an important new weapon to integrate with other treatment modalities such as radiation, chemotherapy, and other drugs.

The most important lesson I learned from my experience with Andrea is to surrender to the mystery of life. We don't know everything. What we now know about healing is only the tip of the mystery. We need to continue to learn, to take lessons from nature continuously, and to understand that we do not have the bottom line. We need to stop and nourish our souls and accept our ignorance and we need to walk the path of discovery. This is the path that I set out upon as my path of destiny in seeking to become a doctor, and then to become an inquiring doctor, probing the boundaries of knowledge through research. At first my probing was directed primarily toward the cause and treatment of disease, ultimately focusing on cancer. The path from there led me to a fork in the road that was prevention.

I remember a comment made by Yogi Berra, who said, "When you get to a fork in the road, take it." I always laughed at that, but then I realized I was exploring two forks of the road in my career as a physician. I treated disease, but the branch in the road led to prevention.

I never dreamed that through my experience with Andrea my eyes would be opened to yet another fork in the road further down. Through the darkness of her illness, bright light shone on the fork that led to complementary medicine, branching out from conventional medicine. Once again, at her urging and because of my love for her, I came to a fork in the road, and I said to myself, "Take it. Don't be afraid. Take the new road and see where it goes."

It is natural for a physician with an open mind, a mind of inquiry, a mind that asks questions and searches out the answers, to explore. To find which forks in the road lead where we want to go, we must go down all of them if they are promising and find new approaches to eradicate the diseases that afflict mankind.

When I look back on my professional career and my personal experiences, what will I think? What do I think now? I think that we are all born with a vision, a mission, some purpose that we must pursue. If we pursue it, at some point down the road we can look back and say mission accomplished. We hope to be able to say we have done at least a small part of what we set out to do.

If we are fortunate, we will learn something more that needs to be accomplished, and so we move ahead. When we move on, we need to move with feelings, purpose, learning, caring for others and ourselves, knowing who we are, and responding to our inner selves, our feelings, and our directions. Feelings, nurturing, spirituality are all part of this process. And as we move on we must see the duality of everything, the good and the bad, life and death. It is all part of the mystery of our existence.

A disease that we see or that we experience or that we help someone through is only one event in the duality of life. The event must not detract from the life but must contribute to the feeling of wholeness. It is the feeling of wholeness that permits healing, perhaps survival, but in any event inner peace. It is inner peace that we all seek but few of us achieve.

I believe that Andrea achieved this inner peace. She was at peace with herself. She felt that her mission in life was to come on to this earth and to have three wonderful children and experience love with them and with me and to experience love herself and to give to the family. She felt she did this. She felt she accomplished her mission in life. In the end she said she would not trade her place with anyone. She was not envious of anyone. She was at peace. Yes, she wanted more time, but for herself, not to become anyone else.

In the end it was love that was the most important thing for her. She felt that and I felt that. Without love there is nothing. Love for another, love for the present, for the moment, love for ourselves and our mission. The experience of love is forever. We all want it to last forever. For Andrea and me, it was a feeling that came from a place of existence that is timeless. It is a feeling that will go on timelessly forever, no matter what physical and spiritual state we are in. We can only journey to other realms of existence from a place of knowing who we are and with love for each other. With love, we can never be separated.

For Further Reading

READERS who have reached this point may also enjoy the following titles.

Andrea's introduction to meditation was *How to Meditate: A Guide to Self-Discovery,* by Dr. Lawrence LeShan. It's available in paperback from Bantam. Among his other books, LeShan's *Cancer as a Turning Point* is published under the Plume imprint.

Dr. Bernie Siegel's *Love, Medicine & Miracles* is available in paperback from Harper Perennial. Siegel's many audio- and videotapes may also be of interest.

Full Catastrophe Living, also now in paperback, from Delta, is Jon Kabat-Zinn's account of how meditation can be used in reducing stress and pain.

Dr. Andrew Weil's *Spontaneous Healing* has already reached many readers. Fawcett Columbine has published the paperback edition currently available.

Bill Moyers's *Healing and the Mind,* first published in 1993 as a companion volume to the popular public television series, brought widespread public attention to explorations in mind-body medicine.

Cancer Free, by me and Dr. Moshe Shike, provides a complete cancer prevention program. It is now available in paperback from Fireside Books.

Susan Sontag's *Illness As Metaphor* has been published in a companion volume with *AIDS and Its Metaphors* by Anchor Books.

Nick Taylor's *A Necessary End,* published by Nan A. Talese/Doubleday in 1994, is an account of coping with the death of his parents.

Norman Cousins's *Anatomy of an Illness* is a classic in the field, and Dr. Sherwin Nuland's *How We Die* is rapidly on its way to becoming one.